41700 (2)

Atlas of Orthopedic Examination of tł

Illustrations by: Kevin Marks

For W. B. Saunders

Editorial Director, Health Sciences: Mary Law
Head of Project Management: Ewan Halley
Project Development Manager: Dinah Thom
Senior Designer: Judith Wright

Atlas of Orthopedic Examination of the Peripheral Joints

Ludwig Ombregt MD

Medical Practitioner in Orthopedic Medicine, Kanegem, Belgium;
International Lecturer in Orthopedic Medicine

Pierre Bisschop

Physiotherapist specializing in Orthopedic Medicine, Knesselare, Belgium;
International Lecturer in Orthopedic Medicine

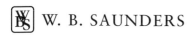 W. B. SAUNDERS

Edinburgh • London • New York • Philadelphia • St Louis • Sydney • Toronto • 1999

W. B. SAUNDERS
An imprint of Harcourt Brace and Company Limited

First published 1999

ISBN 0 7020 2124 5

British Library Cataloguing in Publication Data
A catalogue record for this book is available from the British
Library.

Library of Congress Cataloging in Publication Data
A catalog record for this book is available from the Library
of Congress.

Note
Medical knowledge is constantly changing. As new
information becomes available, changes in treatment,
procedures, equipment and the use of drugs become
necessary. The authors and the publishers have, as far as it is
possible, taken care to ensure that the information given in
this text is accurate and up-to-date. However, readers are
strongly advised to confirm that the information, especially
with regard to drug usage, complies with the latest
legislation and standards of practice.

The
publisher's
policy is to use
**paper manufactured
from sustainable forests**

Printed in China

Contents

Preface

This manuscript was developed as a manual for medical and physiotherapy students. Its purpose is to fill the existing information and training gap between the descriptive anatomy and the pathology of the peripheral joints.

During our courses in orthopedic medicine we are almost daily confronted by postgraduate students (both physiotherapists and doctors) who do not have practical knowledge in topographic, surface and functional anatomy. Despite the fact that all clinical skills start with an understanding of the normal, the study of the clinical appearance of normal tissues and their behaviour during manual examination seems to be a grossly neglected area of medical education.

This book essentially addresses the clinical appearance of normal tissues and their function, and provides guidance on the examination and assessment of normal joints. We confined ourselves to a discussion of the most important tests used in orthopedic medicine. They are relatively simple to perform and have a great inter-tester reliability. These tests (active, passive and resisted movements) are accepted in orthopedic medicine, physiotherapy and manual therapy as the basic tests for a good clinical evaluation of the joint in question. This book focuses on the perfect technical execution of the movements. Much to our regret we have to conclude that poorly conducted tests often give incorrect information and therefore lead to inaccurate diagnoses. We believe that our teaching experience may be of great help to the reader and therefore we have listed the errors students most frequently make in the section on 'common mistakes'.

A small section on 'common pathological situations' follows a discussion of the technical execution of the test, and findings in normal subjects. This section could be confusing in that the described test is not meant to be the diagnostic procedure for the referred condition. A clinical diagnosis does not rely on the outcome of one single test but is made on the interpretation of a clinical pattern (the combined outcome of a set of clinical tests). The interpretation of pathological findings and the building up of clinical patterns is not within the scope of this book. The interested reader is referred to our clinical reference book *A System of Orthopaedic Medicine* published by Saunders in 1995. In this work, all pathological conditions and their conservative treatments are discussed thoroughly.

Acknowledgements

We would like to thank colleagues who are teachers of Orthopaedic Medicine International (OMI) and who provided significant help. We are particularly grateful to Dr Eric Barbaix, Teacher in Manual Therapy at the University of Brussels, who acted as an excellent adviser, providing both expertise and constructive criticism.

The following figures have been taken from Ombregt J, Bisschop P, ter Veer H J, Van de Velde T

1995 A system of orthopaedic medicine. W B Saunders, London: 1.8–1.16, 1.18–1.34; 2.1, 2.3, 2.4, 2.8–2.12, 2.14–2.16, 2.19–2.21, 2.24–2.35; 3.3, 3.4, 3.6, 3.10, 3.11, 3.15, 3.16, 3.18, 3.23, 3.24, 3.27–3.60; 4.5, 4.11, 4.13, 4.14, 4.16–4.20, 4.22–4.32, 4.35, 4.36; 5.6–5.11, 5.14, 5.18, 5.21–5.43, 5.45–5.50; 6.5, 6.10–6.12, 6.16, 6.18, 6.20, 6.24–6.43.

Kanegem-Tielt, 1999   Ludwig Ombregt
                                               Pierre Bisschop

Introduction

The purpose of examination and / or testing procedures in orthopedic medicine is to examine the *function* of the different tissues of the moving parts. The techniques are based on the principle of 'selective tension'.

Each tissue of the body has its particular function. It acts either as an isolated structure or as part of a group of structures. Function differs, depending on whether a tissue is built to make other tissues move (musculo-tendinous structures), to control range of movement (capsulo-ligamentous structures), to facilitate movement (bursae) or to activate movement (nerve structures).

The musculo-tendinous unit has the inherent capability to contract – it is a 'contractile tissue' – whereas all the other structures do not possess this capability – they are 'inert'. Contractile structures can be tested (= put under tension) by provoking a maximal isometric contraction. Inert structures are tested by putting them under maximal stretch.

Active movements

An active movement is performed as far as it may go. It does not follow the principle of 'testing by selective tension': a lot of structures are put under stress. The examiner not only gets an idea of the possible range of motion in the joint (normal, limited or excessive), he is also informed about the integrity of the musculo-tendinous apparatus.

Passive movements

A passive movement brings a joint to the end of the normal range. The normal amplitude differs from the theoretical range of motion. Articular surfaces allow a certain amount of movement, but the movement is usually stopped as a result of tension in the capsulo-ligamentous structures. The movement therefore not only informs the examiner about the normal range, but also about the structures that stop the movement from going further. This happens by assessing the end-feel of a movement which can be either elastic (capsular), hard (bony or ligamentous) or soft (tissue approximation).

Passive movements are good tests to examine the inert structures and give an answer to the following questions:

a. Does the inert structure function normally? If not, pain may be elicited and / or the range may have diminished.
b. Does it allow a normal range of motion? If not, the end-feel will have changed.

From the technical point of view the examiner should position him or herself in such a way that the movemet can be executed over the entire possible range of motion and can be brought to the end of the range in order to test the end-feel. It may be necessary to fixate the subject's body or part of the subject's limb in order to avoid parasitary movements that would give rise to an incorrect answer.

Resisted movements

A resisted movement is meant to test the muscular tissue only. It should be executed in an isometric way, thereby holding the joint in the neutral position: this puts strain on the contractile tissue but leaves the inert structures unattended. The test activates certain muscles or muscle groups (= different muscles with the same function). It informs the examiner about the normal strength of the contraction.

Resisted movements test the contractile structure: the whole of the muscle belly, the musculotendinous junction, the body of the tendon and the insertion onto the bone. When a lesion in one of these parts is present, the contraction will result in pain with or withour weakness. Diminution of strength is the result of either a rupture or of a problem with the nervous system activating the muscle.

The examiner should position him or herself in such a way that he or she is stronger than the subject: the only way to execute the movements in an isometric way. The joint is brought into the neutral position, allowing the inert tissues to relax, and the subject is asked to perform a contraction with maximal strength. The examiner resists the movement, thereby not allowing any articular movement at all. He or she therefore puts his or her hands in such a way that one hand exerts pressure while the other gives counter-pressure.

The correctness of the technical execution of the tests guarantees the correctness of the answer.

Further reading

Daniels L, Worthinghaus C 1995 Muscle testing. Saunders, London

Kapandji I A 1987 The physiology of the joints, vol I. Churchill Livingstone, Edinburgh

Ombregt L, Bisschop P, ter Veer H, Van de Velde A 1995 A system of orthopaedic medicine. Saunders, London

Petty N J, Moore A P 1998 Neuromusculoskeletal examination and assessment: a handbook for therapists. Churchill Livingstone, Edinburgh

1

Shoulder

SURFACE AND PALPATORY ANATOMY

The shoulder is inextricably bound up with the shoulder girdle, anteriorly via the clavicle and at the posterior aspect via the scapula. These two bony structures are easily detectable landmarks to start the palpation of the shoulder structures.

Bony landmarks

Anterolateral (Figs 1.1 and 1.2)

The clavicle (A) is the most prominent bone and is easily detectable because it lies subcutaneously. Its medial part is convex and the lateral third is concave. Its medial end (sternal end) is bulbous and articulates with the sternum.

The lateral end is flattened and articulates with

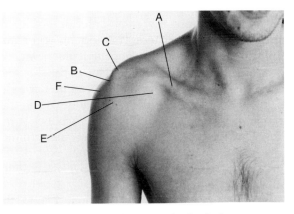

Fig. 1.1   Anterior view of the shoulder (in vivo).

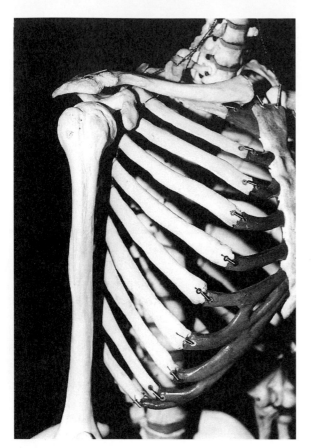

Fig. 1.2 Anterior view of the shoulder (skeleton).

the scapula's acromion (B) which can be recognized as a flat bone overlying the shoulder joint. Palpate the anterior aspect of the clavicle and continue further laterally until the acromial end (C) is felt. Just lateral to it a small indentation is palpable before the clear anterior border of the acromion is reached. This indentation is the anterior end of the acromioclavicular joint. By moving the palpating finger on top of the shoulder the acromial end of the clavicle can be felt to lie slightly higher than the acromion. When the finger lies in contact with the two bones – the clavicle and the acromion – it lies on the acromioclavicular joint of which the upper part of the capsule is reinforced with the superior acromioclavicular ligament.

In the infraclavicular fossa just below the concave lateral part of the clavicle a bony promi-

nence can be felt. This is the scapula's coracoid process (D), of which only the tip and the medial surface are palpable. They form the points of origin for the short head of the biceps brachii muscle and for the coracobrachialis muscle respectively.

Place the finger on the coracoid process and go 1 cm down. Now move the finger laterally until a sharp bony structure is reached. This is the lesser tuberosity (E) of the head of the humerus. Palpate this bone and feel for its lateral border – the medial lip of the intertubercular sulcus.

Just lateral to this border lies the bicipital groove that contains the long head of the biceps. This intertubercular sulcus is palpable with the thumb placed flat on it and during rotatory movements of the humerus. To define the bicipital groove, use the subject's forearm as a lever and rotate the humerus laterally until the medial lip of the sulcus hits the thumb; then rotate the arm medially until the lateral lip catches the thumb.

At the lateral aspect of the sulcus a greater tubercle can be palpated. This is the greater tuberosity (F). When moving the palpating finger upwards a depression can be felt before the lateral border of the acromion is reached.

Posterolateral (Figs 1.3 and 1.4)

The scapula (A) is the most important bone at the posterior side of the thorax. It has a very prominent spine (B) that is easy to palpate. Feel

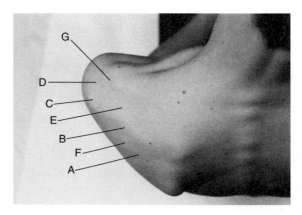

Fig. 1.3 View of the shoulder from above.

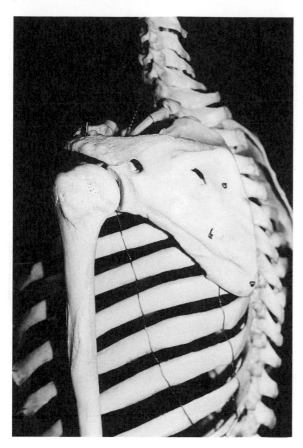

Fig. 1.4 Posterolateral view of the shoulder (skeleton).

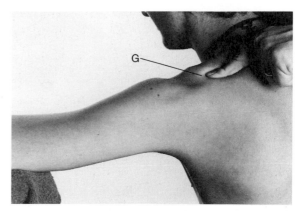

Fig. 1.5 Palpation of the supraspinous fossa (shoulder in abduction).

between the clavicle and acromion. The acromio-clavicular joint line joins these two points.

Palpation of soft tissue

Palpation of the deltoid muscle

The deltoid muscle is easy to recognize. It forms the most important muscular mass of the shoulder and is responsible for its round look (Fig. 1.6). The anterior portion (A) overlies the anterior border of the acromion and the lesser tuberosity. The middle portion (B) lies over the lateral border of the acromion and the greater tuberosity, and the posterior portion (C) builds the posterior aspect of the shoulder and covers the lateral part of the spine of the scapula.

for the posterior margin of the spine and follow this further laterally where it becomes more prominent. The spine can be felt to make a 90° forwards turn – the acromial angle (C) – before it forms the acromion (D). Together with the acromial end of the clavicle and the coracoacromial ligament it forms the coracoacromial roof.

The spine divides the scapula into a supraspinous fossa (E) and an infraspinous fossa (F), in which lie, respectively, the supraspinatus and the infraspinatus muscle bellies.

Place the subject sitting with the arm in 90° abduction and palpate in the supraspinous fossa in a lateral direction. The spine of the scapula is felt to meet the clavicle. At this point lies the posterior aspect of the acromioclavicular joint (G) (Fig. 1.5). Place the thumb at this point and palpate simultaneously for the anterior indentation

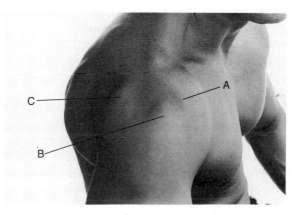

Fig. 1.6 Lateral view of the shoulder (in vivo).

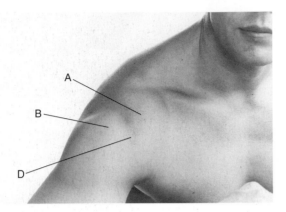

Fig. 1.7 View of the deltoid muscle (during contraction).

Ask the subject to abduct the arm against resistance. A groove (D) (Fig. 1.7) can be palpated between the anterior and middle portions of the deltoid. This overlies the bicipital groove.

Palpation of the supraspinatus muscle

Muscle belly and musculotendinous junction. The subject sits with the arm in full abduction and rested on the couch. The elbow now lies on the same level as the shoulder. The examiner stands behind the subject. The trapezius muscle is well relaxed and palpation can be performed through that muscle. Palpate for the spine of the scapula. The muscle belly lying just above the spine of the scapula is the supraspinatus muscle. It fills up the supraspinous fossa. Move the palpating finger more laterally until it reaches the corner formed between the clavicle and the spine of the scapula. The finger now lies on the musculotendinous junction of the supraspinatus, which can be felt to continue laterally under the acromion (Fig. 1.8).

Insertion on the greater tuberosity. Now position the subject with the forearm behind the back. The arm is now in full internal rotation. Palpate for the lateral border of the acromion; follow it in the anterior direction until the corner is felt between the lateral and anterior border and identify the latter. Also look for the acromioclavicular joint and keep the palpating finger lateral to it. Move the finger forwards so that it comes to lie on the

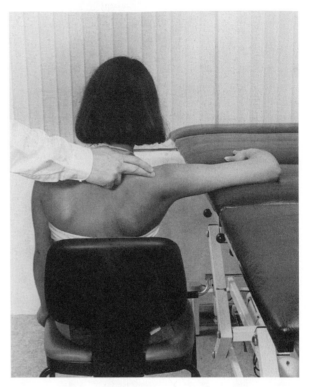

Fig. 1.8 Palpation of the musculotendinous junction of the supraspinatus.

greater tuberosity of the humerus but is still in contact with the acromion as well. Exert a pressure vertically downwards against the humerus. The finger now lies on the supraspinatus tendon of which the medial border can be felt quite clearly (Fig. 1.9).

Palpation of the infraspinatus muscle (Fig. 1.10). The subject is in prone lying and rests on the elbows. The upper arm should be kept vertical and in slight adduction. The subject therefore leans towards the shoulder to be palpated. With the hand he grasps the edge of the couch. This results in some external rotation of the shoulder as well. The examiner looks for the spine of the scapula and palpates below it, in the infraspinous fossa. The thumb now lies on the infraspinatus muscle belly. Place the thumb just under the spine of scapula and palpate more and more laterally. A tendon will be felt that runs parallel to this spine. This is the infraspinatus tendon.

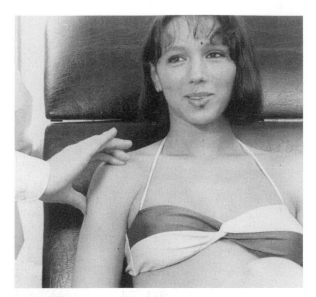

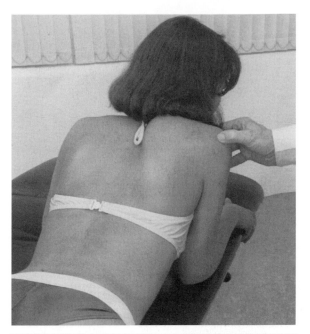

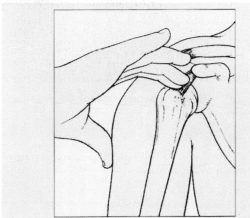

Fig. 1.9 Palpation of the tenoperiosteal junction of the supraspinatus.

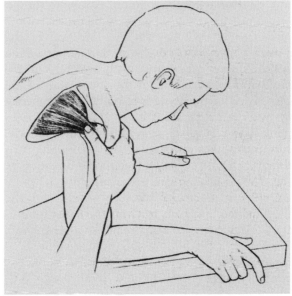

It can be followed until the attachment on the greater tuberosity is found. The bone can be felt through the tendinous mass. Palpate more laterally until the thumb lies on the greater tuberosity. The tendinous structure cannot be felt any more. Come back to the previous point where both bone and tendon are felt. This is the insertion.

Palpation of the subscapularis tendon

The subscapularis muscle belly can only be reached by bringing the hand in between the

Fig. 1.10 Palpation of the tenoperiosteal junction of the infraspinatus.

scapula and the thorax. It cannot really be palpated. The tendinous insertion on the lesser tuberosity, however, can easily be palpated.

The subject is in a half lying position on a couch, the upper arm along the body and the elbow flexed to 90°. The examiner grasps the

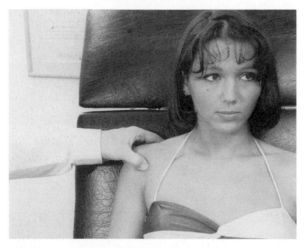

Fig. 1.11 Pushing the tendons of the short head of biceps and of coracobrachialis medially.

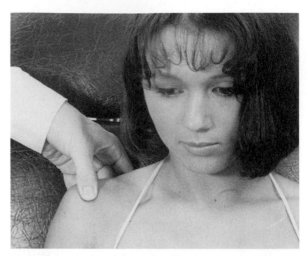

Fig. 1.12 Palpation of the subscapularis (upper part).

subject's hand and brings the shoulder into a few degrees external rotation. Place the thumb of the other hand on the lesser tuberosity of the humerus. It now lies on the insertion of the subscapularis tendon. The contact is not direct, because the insertion is partly covered by, on the one hand, the tendons of the short head of the biceps and of the coracobrachialis, both running towards the coracoid process and, on the other hand, the anterior portion of the deltoid muscle, running in the direction of the acromion. Turn the thumb so that its tip lies in the direction of the xiphoid process of the sternum (Fig. 1.11).

Push the muscular mass forwards, flex the thumb and come back towards the lesser tuberosity. The two tendons can be felt snapping away. They now lie medially to the thumb. At the same time, deltoid fibres have been drawn sideways and lie laterally to the thumb, which now is in direct contact with the subscapularis insertion (Figs 1.12 and 1.13).

Palpation of the long head of biceps (Fig. 1.14)

Place the finger in the groove between the anterior and middle portions of the deltoid muscle. Move the finger anteriorly and distally. It now lies on the bicipital groove, which is situated more laterally than is usually supposed.

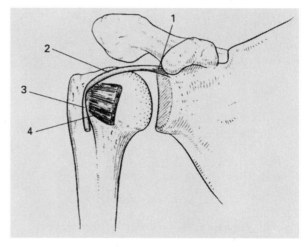

Fig. 1.13 Anterior view of the shoulder: 1, glenoid insertion of the biceps; 2 and 3, biceps tendon; 4, insertion of the subscapularis muscle.

Identify the intertubercular sulcus by placing the thumb flat on it and by executing small rotatory movements of the humerus. The lateral and medial lips can be felt catching against the thumb. In this groove lies the tendon of the long head of biceps. It is difficult to palpate as it is covered with a transverse ligament. Move the thumb upwards until the upper part of the groove is reached, just below the acromion. Ask for

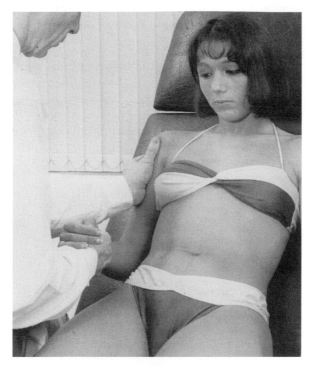

Fig. 1.14 Palpation of the long head of biceps in the sulcus.

an active flexion of the elbow and resist the movement. Tightening of the tendon can be felt.

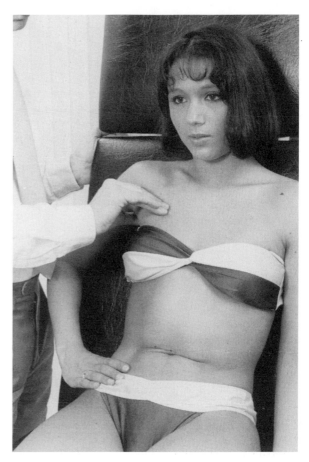

Fig. 1.15 Palpation of the muscle belly of the pectoralis major.

Palpation of the pectoralis major muscle
(Fig. 1.15)

The lateral aspect of the pectoralis major muscle forms the anterior border of the axilla where its inferior border can be palpated very well, especially during resisted adduction of the arm. The tendon inserts at the crest of the greater tuberosity, just below the lateral border of the bicipital sulcus.

Palpation of the latissimus dorsi muscle
(Fig. 1.16)

The lateral aspect of the latissimus dorsi muscle builds the posterior border of the axilla. It is felt to contract during resisted adduction of the arm. Its insertion lies anteriorly at the crest of the lesser tuberosity.

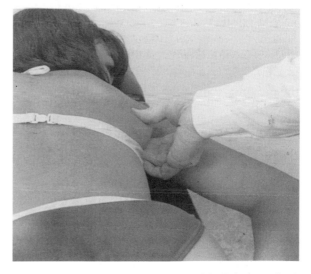

Fig. 1.16 Palpation of the axillar part of the latissimus dorsi.

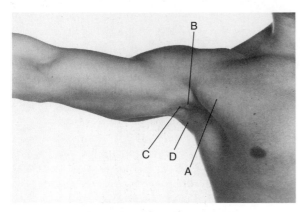

Fig. 1.17 Anterior view of the axilla.

Palpation of the axilla

Bring the subject's arm into 90° abduction. Ask him to press the arm downwards and resist this movement. During palpation in the antero-posterior direction the following structures can be identified (Fig. 1.17): pectoralis major (A), forming the anterior border of the axilla, the tendon of the short head of biceps (B), the coraco-brachialis muscle (C), and the latissimus dorsi (D), forming the posterior border.

FUNCTIONAL EXAMINATION OF THE SHOULDER

Introduction/general remarks

Shoulder lesions give rise to pain felt mostly in the proximal part of the upper limb. The shoulder examination is therefore commonly used in the diagnosis of upper arm pain. However, the examiner should realize that symptoms in the region of the shoulder can also originate from the cervical spine, the upper thoracic spine and the shoulder girdle. The examination of the shoulder is to be considered as an element in the diagnostic procedures for lesions of the upper quadrant.

ACTIVE TEST

Active elevation

Positioning. The subject stands with the arms hanging alongside the body. The examiner stands behind.

Procedure. Ask the subject to bring up both arms sideways as high as possible (Fig. 1.18).

Common mistakes:
- The movement is not performed to the very end of the possible range.
- The arms are brought up in a sagittal plane.
- The arms are kept in internal rotation, which makes full movement impossible.

Normal functional anatomy:
- *Range*: 180°
- *Structures involved*: Many structures are committed. The movement is started by the supraspinatus muscle and continued by the

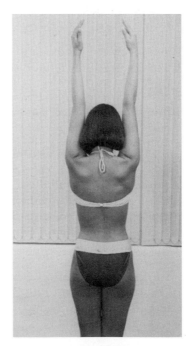

Fig. 1.18 Active elevation of the arm.

middle portion of the deltoid and by the long head of biceps. Rotation of the scapula is done mainly by the serratus anterior muscle, supported by the trapezius muscle, especially towards the end of range. The movement also stretches and/or squeezes several structures, such as the capsule of the glenohumeral joint, the subdeltoid bursa, and the sternoclavicular and acromioclavicular ligaments.

Meaning. This a very non-specific test, which is almost always disturbed when a shoulder or shoulder girdle pathology is present. It also gives an idea of the patient's willingness to cooperate.

Pain at mid-range may indicate a structure in between the humeral head and the coracoacromial arch – either one of the tendons of supraspinatus, infraspinatus, subscapularis, long head of biceps, or the subacromial bursa or inferior acromio-clavicular ligament – being painfully pinched. The patient often avoids painful impingement by adding an anterior component over part of the movement.

Limitation with or without pain occurs in shoulder arthritis or arthrosis, in certain extra-capsular lesions and in some neurological conditions causing weakness of the shoulder elevators.

PASSIVE TESTS

Passive elevation

Positioning. The subject stands with the arms hanging alongside the body. The examiner stands behind the subject and takes hold of the elbow at the distal part of the upper arm.

Procedure. Take the arm up sideways in the frontal plane as far as possible. Allow some external rotation about 90° of abduction. Reaching the end of range, give counter-pressure with the other hand at the subject's opposite shoulder (Fig. 1.19).

Common mistakes:
- When the arm is grasped distally to the subject's elbow, elbow movement prevents assessment of end-feel.
- The arm is not allowed to externally rotate.

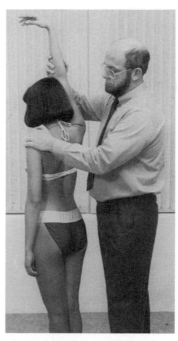

Fig. 1.19 Passive elevation of the arm.

- The movement is stopped before the end of the possible range is reached.
- At the end of range the arm is taken backwards in a sagittal plane.
- Insufficient counter-pressure results in the subject side-flexing the body.

Normal functional anatomy:
- *Range*: 180°
- *End-feel*: elastic
- *Limiting structures*:
  - the axillary part of the joint capsule
  - stretching of the acromioclavicular and sternoclavicular ligaments
  - the adductors and internal rotators of the shoulder
  - contact between the lesser tuberosity of the humerus and the upper part of the glenoid labrum.

Common pathological situations:
- The movement can be painful in subdeltoid bursitis and in rotator cuff tendinitis, as well as in acromioclavicular lesions.

- Limitation occurs in arthritis and arthrosis of the shoulder and in serious extracapsular conditions.

Passive external rotation

Positioning. The subject stands with the upper arm alongside the body and the elbow flexed to a right angle. The examiner stands level with the subject's arm and stabilizes the elbow with his trunk. One hand is placed on the contralateral shoulder to stabilize the shoulder girdle and trunk; the other takes hold of the distal forearm.

Procedure. Rotate the arm outwards, meanwhile assuring the vertical position of the humerus, until the movement comes to an elastic stop (Fig. 1.20).

Common mistakes:
- The shoulder girdle is not well enough fixed so that trunk movement is allowed to happen.
- The elbow is not well stabilized so that shoulder abduction or extension occurs.
- The movement is not performed to the end of the possible range.

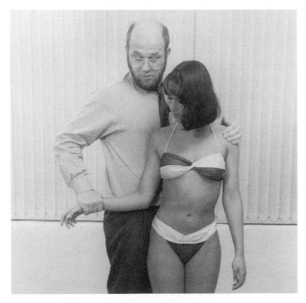

Fig. 1.20 Passive external rotation test for the glenohumeral joint.

Normal functional anatomy:
- *Range*: 90°
- *End-feel*: elastic
- *Limiting structures*:
  - the anterior portion of the joint capsule
  - the internal rotator muscles of the shoulder
  - contact between the greater tuberosity of the humerus and the posterior part of the glenoid labrum.

Common pathological situations:
- Pain on full passive external rotation is one of the first signs of shoulder arthritis. External rotation also stretches the acromioclavicular ligaments and the subscapularis tendon, and squeezes the subdeltoid bursa.
- Isolated limitation occurs in contracture of the anterior capsule and in subcoracoid bursitis.
- The movement is markedly limited as part of a capsular pattern of limitation of movement in moderate or more advanced arthritis. Depending on the condition being either acute or chronic, the end-feel will be either of muscle spasm or hard.
- Excessive range may indicate shoulder instability.

Passive external rotation with the shoulder in 90° abduction

Positioning. The subject stands with the arm hanging alongside the body and the elbow flexed to 90°. The examiner stands level with the subject's arm. The contralateral hand takes hold of the elbow and brings the arm into 90° of abduction. The other hand grasps the distal forearm.

Procedure. Put the shoulder into external rotation, meanwhile stabilizing the elbow (Fig. 1.21).

Common mistakes. If the movement is too painful the patient will move the body backwards.

Normal functional anatomy:
- *Range*: 90°
- *End-feel*: elastic
- *Limiting structures*:
  - the anterior part of the joint capsule

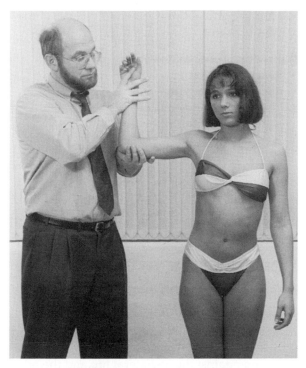

Fig. 1.21   Passive horizontal external rotation.

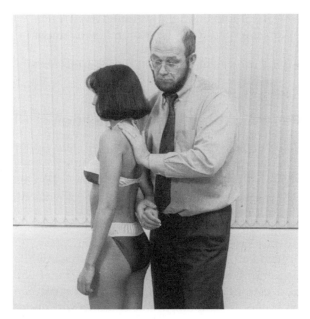

Fig. 1.22   Passive internal rotation test for the glenohumeral joint.

   – the adductors and internal rotators of the shoulder.

Common pathological situations:
- The movement is limited in arthritis and arthrosis of the shoulder and also in isolated contracture of the anterior part of the joint capsule.
- Excessive movement may be present in shoulder instability.

Passive internal rotation

Positioning. The subject stands with the upper arm alongside the body and the elbow flexed to a right angle. The examiner stands level with the subject's arm and stabilizes the elbow with his trunk. One hand is placed on the opposite shoulder to stabilize the shoulder girdle and trunk; the other takes hold of the distal forearm.

Procedure. Bring the subject's forearm behind her back and move her hand away from her body as far as possible (Fig. 1.22).

Common mistakes:
- The shoulder is held in too much abduction.
- The elbow is pulled backwards, which creates an extension of the shoulder instead of internal rotation.
- The hand is moved upwards instead of backwards.

Normal functional anatomy:
- *Range*: 90°
- *End-feel*: elastic
- *Limiting structures*:
   – the posterior part of the joint capsule
   – the external rotator muscles of the shoulder
   – contact between the lesser tuberosity of the humerus and the anterior part of the glenoid labrum of the scapula.

Common pathological situations:
- Pain at the end of range may occur in lesions of the infraspinatus and supraspinatus tendons, and also of the acromioclavicular ligaments.
- Pain at mid-range may occur in rotator cuff tendinitis or in subacromial bursitis.

- More or less limitation is found as part of a capsular pattern of limitation of movement in moderate and severe arthritis.
- Excessive range may indicate shoulder instability.

Passive glenohumeral abduction

Positioning. The subject stands with the upper arm alongside the body. The examiner stands level with and behind the subject's arm. One hand takes hold of the elbow, just above the joint. The thumb of the other hand is placed against the lateral aspect of the lower angle of the scapula.

Procedure. Abduct the arm slowly, meanwhile preventing the scapula from moving (Fig. 1.23). End of range is reached when the scapula can no longer be stabilized and starts to slip under the thumb.

Common mistakes:
- The scapula is not stabilized sufficiently.
  - *Alternative technique*: When the lower angle of the scapula cannot be stabilized, the lateral margin may be used. The scapula can also be stabilized by placing one hand upon the acromion.

- Movement is not performed to the end of the possible range.

Normal functional anatomy:
- *Range*: 90°
- *End-feel*: ligamentous
- *Limiting structures*:
  - the axillary part of the joint capsule
  - contact between the greater tuberosity and the upper part of the glenoid labrum.

Common pathological situations:
- The movement is limited in shoulder arthritis.
- It may also become restricted in acute subdeltoid bursitis.

ISOMETRIC CONTRACTIONS
Resisted adduction

Positioning. The subject stands with the arm hanging and slightly abducted. The examiner stands level with the subject's arm. He places one hand against the ipsilateral hip and the other hand against the inner aspect of the elbow.

Procedure. Resist the subject's attempt to adduct her arm (Fig. 1.24).

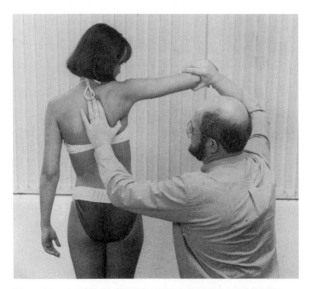

Fig. 1.23 Passive scapulohumeral abduction test for the glenohumeral joint.

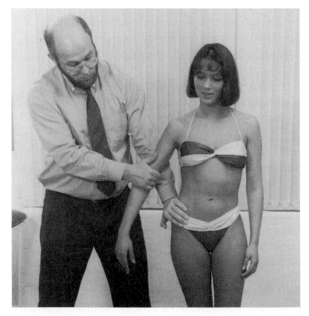

Fig. 1.24 Resisted adduction of the shoulder.

Common mistakes:
- The elbow is allowed to flex.
- Movement is allowed at the shoulder.

Anatomical structures tested:

Muscle function:
- *Important adductors*:
  - Pectoralis major
  - Latissimus dorsi
  - Teres major
  - Teres minor
- *Less important adductors*:
  - Long head of triceps brachii
  - Short head of biceps brachii
  - Clavicular part of deltoid
  - Spinal part of deltoid.

Neural function:

Muscle	Innervation	
	Peripheral	Nerve root
Pectoralis major	Pectoral	C5–C8
Latissimus dorsi	Thoracodorsal	(C6), C7, (C8)
Teres major	Subscapular	C5–C8
Teres minor	Axillary	C5, (C6)
Triceps brachii	Radial	(C6), C7, (C8)
Biceps brachii	Musculocutaneous	C5, C6
Deltoid	Axillary	C5, (C6)
spinal part	Axillary	C5, (C6)
clavicular part	Pectoral	C5–C8

Common pathological situations:
- Pain suggests a lesion in one of the adductor muscles or in the thoracic wall.
- Weakness occurs in severe C7 nerve root palsy.
- Painful weakness is perceived in rib fractures and more rarely in a rupture of the pectoralis major muscle.

Resisted abduction

Positioning. The subject stands with the arm hanging and slightly abducted. The examiner stands level with the subject's arm. He places one hand against the opposite hip and the other hand against the outer aspect of the elbow.

Procedure. Resist the subject's attempt to abduct the arm (Fig. 1.25).

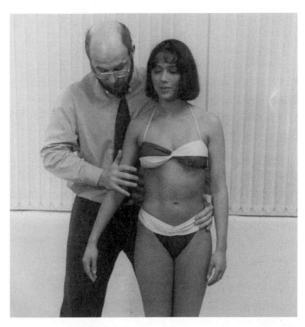

Fig. 1.25 Resisted abduction of the shoulder.

Common mistakes. Movement is allowed at the shoulder.

Anatomical structures tested:

Muscle function:
- *Important abductors*:
  - Deltoid
  - Supraspinatus
- *Less important abductors*:
  - Long head of biceps brachii.

Neural function:

Muscle	Innervation	
	Peripheral	Nerve root
Deltoid	Axillary	C5, (C6)
Supraspinatus	Suprascapular	C5, (C6)
Biceps brachii	Musculocutaneous	C5, C6

Common pathological situations:
- Pain is usually the result of a supraspinatus tendinitis, more rarely of a lesion of the deltoid, but may also occur in subdeltoid bursitis.
- Weakness occurs in total rupture of the

supraspinatus tendon or in neurological conditions, such as lesions of the axillary nerve, the suprascapular nerve or the C5 nerve root.

• Painful weakness is indicative of a recent partial rupture of the supraspinatus tendon.

Resisted external rotation

Positioning. The subject stands with the upper arm against the body and the elbow flexed to a right angle. The forearm is held in the sagittal plane, so keeping the shoulder in a neutral position. The examiner stands level with the subject's arm. He places one hand on the opposite shoulder and the other hand against the outer and distal aspect of the forearm, which he supports.

Procedure. Ask the subject to keep the elbow against the trunk and resist the attempt to push the hand laterally (Fig. 1.26).

Common mistakes. The subject tends to execute the test wrongly either by bringing the shoulder

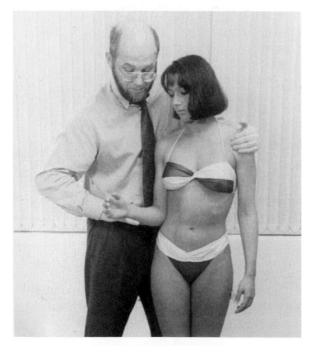

Fig. 1.26 Resisted external rotation of the shoulder.

into abduction or by extending the elbow, especially when weakness is present.

Anatomical structures tested:

Muscle function:
• *Important external rotators*:
  – Infraspinatus
  – Teres minor
• *Less important external rotators*:
  – Spinal part of deltoid.

Neural function:

Muscle	Innervation	
	Peripheral	Nerve root
Infraspinatus	Suprascapular	C5, (C6)
Teres minor	Axillary	C5, (C6)
Deltoid	Axillary	C5, (C6)

Common pathological situations:
• Pain occurs in infraspinatus tendinitis but may also be present in subdeltoid bursitis.
• Weakness indicates a total rupture of the infraspinatus tendon or a neurological condition, e.g. C5 nerve root palsy, suprascapular nerve palsy, neuralgic amyotrophy. Bilateral weakness is suggestive of myopathy.
• Painful weakness is the result of a partial rupture of the infraspinatus tendon.

Resisted internal rotation

Positioning. The subject stands with the upper arm against the body and the elbow flexed to a right angle. The forearm is held in the sagittal plane, so keeping the shoulder in a neutral position. The examiner stands level with the subject's arm. He places one hand on the opposite shoulder and the other hand against the inner and distal aspect of the forearm.

Procedure. Resist the subject's attempt to pull her hand towards her (Fig. 1.27).

Common mistakes:
• The shoulder is allowed to abduct.
• Movement is allowed at the shoulder.

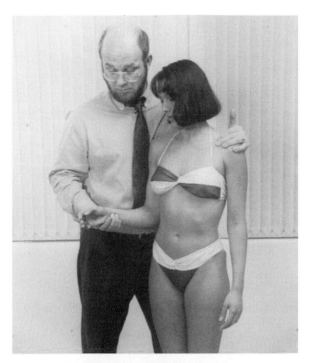

Fig. 1.27 Resisted internal rotation of the shoulder.

Anatomical structures tested:

Muscle function:
* *Important internal rotators:*
  – Subscapularis
  – Pectoralis major
  – Latissimus dorsi
  – Teres major
* *Less important internal rotators:*
  – Long head of biceps brachii
  – Clavicular part of deltoid

Neural function:

Muscle	Innervation	
	Peripheral	Nerve root
Subscapularis	Subscapular	C5–C8
Pectoralis major	Pectoral	C5–C8
Latissimus dorsi	Thoracodorsal	(C6), C7, (C8)
Teres major	Subscapular	C5–C8
Biceps brachii	Musculocutaneous	C5, C6
Deltoid		
clavicular part	Pectoral	C5–C8

Common pathological situations:
* Pain is the result of a lesion of the subscapularis, pectoralis major or latissimus dorsi tendons or muscles, and more rarely of the teres major.
* Isolated weakness occurs in total rupture of the subscapularis tendon.

Resisted flexion of the elbow

Positioning. The subject stands with the arm alongside the body, the elbow bent to a right angle and the forearm in full supination. The examiner stands level with the subject's hand. One hand is on top of the shoulder and the other on the distal aspect of the forearm.

Procedure. Resist the subject's attempt to flex her elbow (Fig. 1.28).

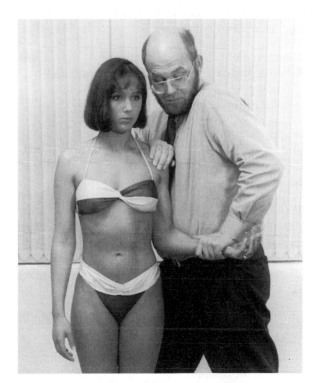

Fig. 1.28 Resisted flexion of the elbow.

Common mistakes:
- The subject shrugs up the shoulder in the hope of exerting more strength.
- Movement is allowed at the elbow.
- In strong subjects, flexion cannot sufficiently be resisted if the resistance is not given perpendicular to the subject's forearm.

Anatomical structures tested:

Muscle function:
- *Important flexors*:
  - Brachialis
  - Biceps brachii
- *Less important flexor*:
  - Brachioradialis.

Neural function:

Muscle	Innervation	
	Peripheral	Nerve root
Brachialis	Musculocutaneous (radial)	C5–C6
Biceps brachii	Musculocutaneous	C5–C6
Brachioradialis	Radial	C5–C6

Common pathological situations:
- Pain in the region of the shoulder occurs when a lesion is present in either the long head or the short head of biceps.
- Weakness is the result of either a C5 or a C6 nerve root lesion.

Resisted extension of the elbow

Positioning. The subject stands with the arm alongside the body and the elbow bent to a right angle with the forearm in supination. The examiner stands level with the subject's forearm. One hand is on top of the shoulder, the other on the distal aspect of the forearm.

Procedure. Resist the subject's attempt to extend the elbow (Fig. 1.29).

Common mistakes:
- Extension is allowed at the shoulder.
- Movement is allowed at the elbow.

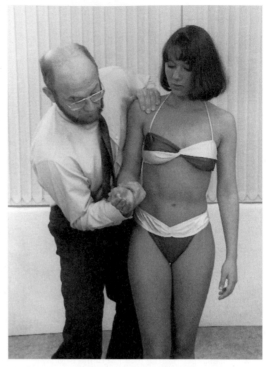

Fig. 1.29 Resisted extension of the elbow.

Anatomical structures tested:

Muscle function:
- *Most important extensor*:
  - Triceps brachii
- *Less important extensor*:
  - Anconeus.

Neural function:

Muscle	Innervation	
	Peripheral	Nerve root
Triceps brachii	Radial	C7–C8
Anconeus	Radial	C7–C8

Common pathological situations:
- Pain elicited in the shoulder region is the result of the humerus being pulled upwards against the acromial arch and pinching an inflamed subacromial structure. This happens in subdeltoid bursitis or in tendinitis of one of the tendons of the rotator cuff.

- Pain on extension more rarely indicates triceps tendinitis.
- Weakness is usually the result of a C7 nerve root palsy.

SPECIFIC TESTS
Passive horizontal adduction

Significance. This test stresses the acromioclavicular and sternoclavicular joints and ligaments. It also squeezes the subcoracoid bursa and the upper part of the insertion of the subscapularis tendon into the lesser tuberosity of the humerus.

Positioning. The subject stands with the arms hanging alongside the body. The examiner stands level with the subject's arm. One hand grasps the elbow at the distal part of the upper arm. The other hand is placed at the back of the other shoulder.

Procedure. Take the arm into abduction first and then bring it horizontally in front of the body, pressing the elbow towards the contralateral shoulder (Fig. 1.30).

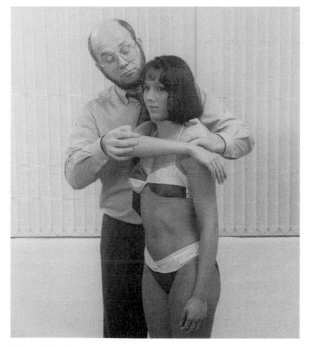

Fig. 1.30 Passive horizontal adduction of the shoulder.

Apprehension test in external rotation

Significance. The test is performed to detect recurrent anterior dislocation of the shoulder. The test is positive when the patient gets the feeling that the shoulder moves out of place, so recognizing her symptoms.

Positioning. The subject lies supine with the arm alongside the body and the elbow flexed to 90°. The examiner sits level with the subject's shoulder. One hand is on the subject's shoulder with the fingers anteriorly and the thumb posteriorly against the humeral head. The other hand takes hold of the forearm.

Procedure. Bring the subject's arm into full external rotation, meanwhile exerting an anterior pressure on the humerus with the thumb (Fig. 1.31). Repeat this test in different degrees of abduction.

Apprehension test in internal rotation

Significance. The test is performed to detect recurrent posterior dislocation of the shoulder. The test is positive when the patient gets the feeling that the shoulder moves out of place, so recognizing her symptoms.

Positioning. The subject sits on a chair, the arm in slight abduction and the forearm behind the back. The examiner sits level with the subject's shoulder. One hand is on the subject's shoulder with the thumb anteriorly and the fingers posteriorly against the humeral head. The other hand grasps the forearm.

Procedure. Bring the subject's arm into slight abduction and full internal rotation and exert a posterior pressure to the humerus with the thumb (Fig. 1.32).

Common mistakes. The subject's shoulder girdle is not well stabilized so that she may twist away from the pressure.

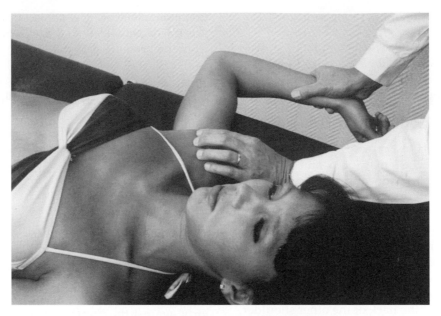

Fig. 1.31   The apprehension test for recurrent anterior dislocation.

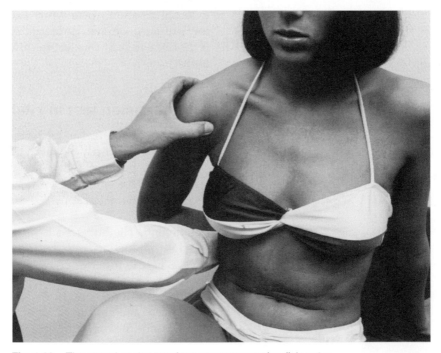

Fig. 1.32   The apprehension test for recurrent posterior dislocation.

Anterior drawer test

Significance. This test is meant to detect anterior hypermobility in the glenohumeral joint.

Positioning. The subject lies supine on the couch with the arm beyond the edge. The examiner stands level with the shoulder. He stabilizes the scapula with the contralateral hand, the thumb of which is placed on the coracoid process and the fingers on the acromion. The arm is brought into about 20° of abduction and into slight flexion.

The forearm is squeezed between the examiner's trunk and the ipsilateral arm, the hand of which grasps the humerus in the axilla (Fig. 1.33).

Procedure. The humeral head is first brought into its neutral position in the glenoid fossa ('loaded') and then glided in the anterior direction.

Posterior drawer test

Significance. This test is meant to detect posterior hypermobility in the glenohumeral joint.

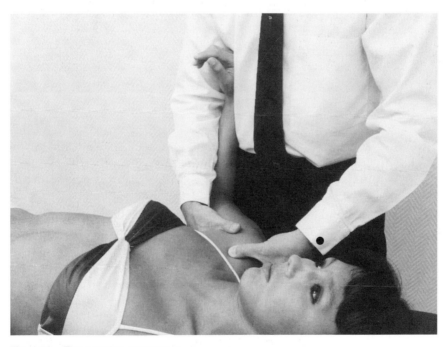

Fig. 1.33   The anterior drawer test.

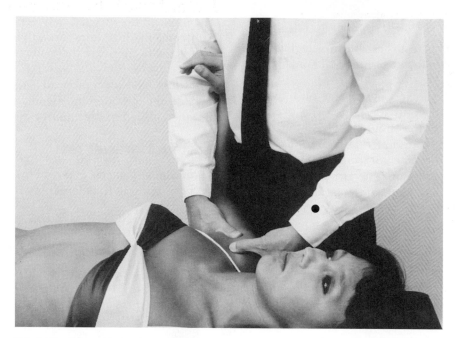

Fig. 1.34   The posterior drawer test.

Positioning. The subject lies supine on the couch with the arm beyond the edge. The examiner stands level with the shoulder. He stabilizes the scapula with the contralateral hand, the thumb of which is placed on the coracoid process and the fingers on the acromion. The arm is brought into about 20° of abduction and into slight flexion. The forearm is squeezed between the examiner's trunk and the ipsilateral arm, the hand of which grasps the humerus in the axilla (Fig. 1.34).

Procedure. The humeral head is first brought into its neutral position in the glenoid fossa ('loaded') and then glided in the posterior direction and slightly laterally.

2

Elbow

SURFACE AND PALPATORY ANATOMY

ANTERIOR

Bony landmarks

There are no real bony landmarks recognizable at the anterior aspect of the elbow. Identify the cubital fossa. Just below it and deeply through the muscles of the anterior and upper part of the forearm, palpate laterally for the radial head (1), and medially for the coronoid process of the ulna (2) (Fig. 2.1). These bony parts can be identified more easily when considering the lateral and medial aspects of the elbow (see below).

Palpation of soft tissue

Palpation of the biceps muscle and the neurovascular structures in the cubital fossa

Keep the subject's elbow slightly flexed. Ask for an active flexion and palpate meanwhile in the cubital fossa with a pinching grip. Feel for the bicipital tendon (Fig. 2.2, A) as an outstanding taut structure. It runs distally to attach to the radial tuberosity. Medial to the tendon its aponeurosis (B) can be felt, and lateral to the tendon the belly of the brachioradialis muscle (C). Proximally the biceps broadens and its musculotendinous junction (D) can be perceived, and even more proximally its muscle belly (Fig. 2.3 and Fig. 2.2, E). Medial to the bicipital tendon, deep under the aponeurosis, lie the brachial artery and the

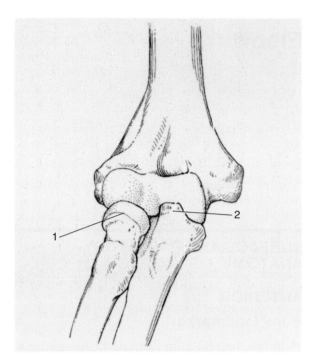

Fig. 2.1 Anterior view of the elbow (skeleton).

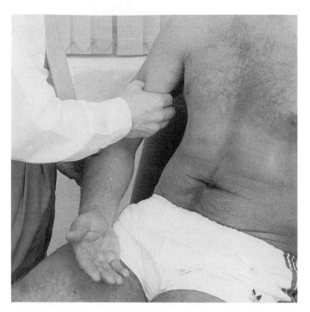

Fig. 2.3 Palpation of the biceps muscle belly.

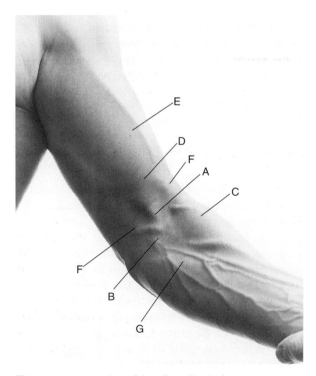

Fig. 2.2 Anterior view of the elbow (in vivo).

median nerve. The former is pulsating, the latter a round strand.

Palpation of the brachialis muscle

Ask the subject to contract the biceps. Place the thumb and fingers in the indentations on both sides of the bicipital tendon (the lateral and medial bicipital grooves) and now ask for an isometric flexion. Under the fingers – and behind the biceps tendon – the contraction of the brachialis muscle (F) can be felt. During relaxation of this muscle, its belly, which runs further distally than the muscle belly of the biceps, can be palpated with a pinching grip. The brachialis inserts at the ulnar tuberosity.

Palpation of the pronator teres muscle

The subject holds his elbow in 90° flexion and the forearm in the neutral position between pronation and supination. Ask the subject to pronate the forearm and resist the movement. Palpate with the other hand in the thick muscular mass

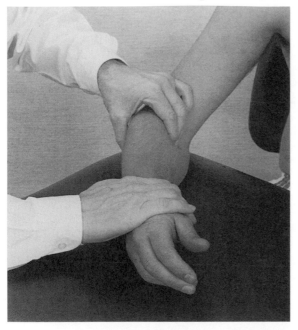

Fig. 2.4   Palpation of the pronator teres muscle.

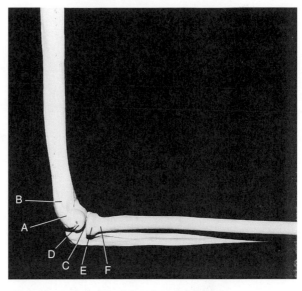

Fig. 2.5   Lateral view of the elbow (skeleton).

just distal to the cubital fossa (Fig. 2.4). A round and strong muscle can be felt running from the medial epicondyle to mid-radius. This is the pronator teres muscle (G).

LATERAL

Bony landmarks (Fig. 2.5)

The subject holds his elbow in 90° of flexion and the forearm supinated. The lateral epicondyle (A) can be palpated as the most prominent bone. From its anterior aspect originates the extensor carpi radialis brevis muscle. The epicondylar border continues proximally in the lateral supracondylar ridge (B). Level with it and from the anterior surface of the humerus originate the brachioradialis and, just below it, the extensor carpi radialis longus muscles.

Palpate distal to the epicondyle for a depression – the radiohumeral joint line (C). Its proximal component – the lateral edge of the humeral capitulum (D) – can be felt as a spherical structure.

The distal component – the head of the radius (E) – is well perceivable when small rotatory movements of the forearm are performed. The joint line becomes a bit wider and thus even better palpable when the elbow is brought towards more extension. Feel for the lower border of the head of the radius and place the finger just distally to it. It now lies on the radial neck (F).

Palpation of soft tissue

Palpation of the brachioradialis muscle (Fig. 2.6)

The subject's elbow is held in 90° flexion and the forearm in the neutral position between pronation and supination. Ask the subject to flex the elbow and resist the movement. The contraction of the brachioradialis muscle (A) is well palpable and visible and the structure can, by palpation in the posterior direction, easily be followed further proximally in its course until its insertion at the anterior aspect of the humerus, level with the lateral supracondylar ridge.

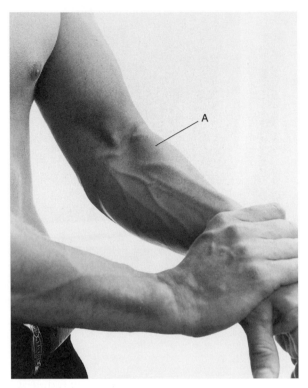

Fig. 2.6 View of the brachioradialis muscle.

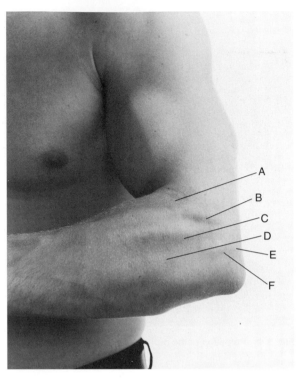

Fig. 2.7 Lateral view of the elbow (in vivo).

Palpation of the radial extensors of the wrist (Fig. 2.7)

The muscles are now relaxed. Bring the subject's forearm into supination and ask him to do a combined active movement of extension and radial deviation of the wrist. Just distal to the origin of the brachioradialis muscle (A) – between this muscle and the lateral epicondyle – the contraction of the extensor carpi radialis longus (B) can be seen. By pressing in the posterior direction, its origin can be palpated, again at the anterior aspect of the humerus (Fig. 2.8).

Go more distally and palpate now the anterior aspect of the lateral epicondyle (E). A flat tendinous structure is recognized which is the origin of the extensor carpi radialis brevis muscle (Fig. 2.9 and Fig. 2.7, C).

Bring the subject's elbow into more extension (130–135°) and into pronation. Over the head of the radius (F) the tendons of wrist and finger extensors (Fig. 2.10 and Fig. 2.7, D) can be palpated.

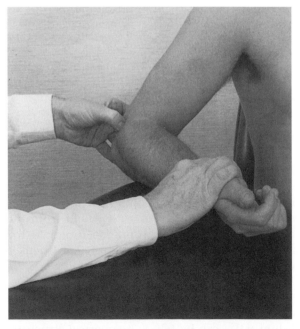

Fig. 2.8 Palpation of the extensor carpi radialis longus muscle.

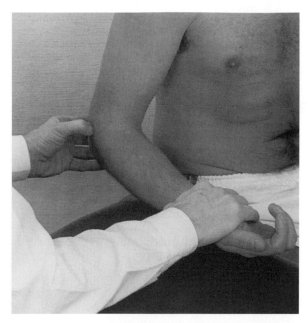
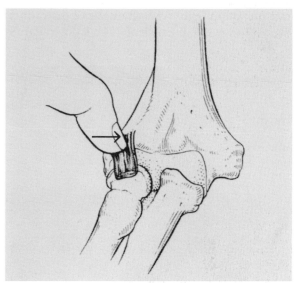

Fig. 2.9   Palpation of the extensor carpi radialis brevis muscle.

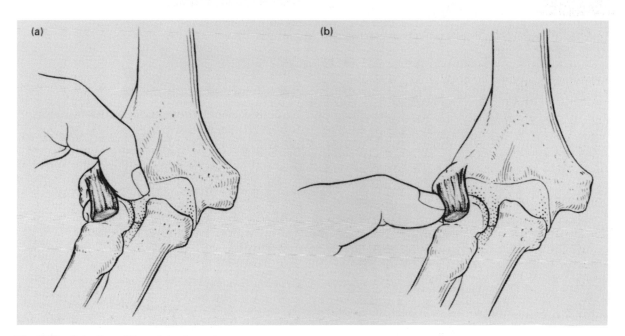

Fig. 2.10   Palpation of the wrist extensors.

Elbow and forearm are again brought into 90° flexion and supination. Use a pinching grip and start palpation level with the neck of the radius (Fig. 2.11). Over a distance of 3–4 cm downwards the bellies of brachioradialis (superficial) and extensors carpi radialis longus and brevis (deep) (Fig. 2.12) can be felt, the latter especially when the subject actively extends his wrist.

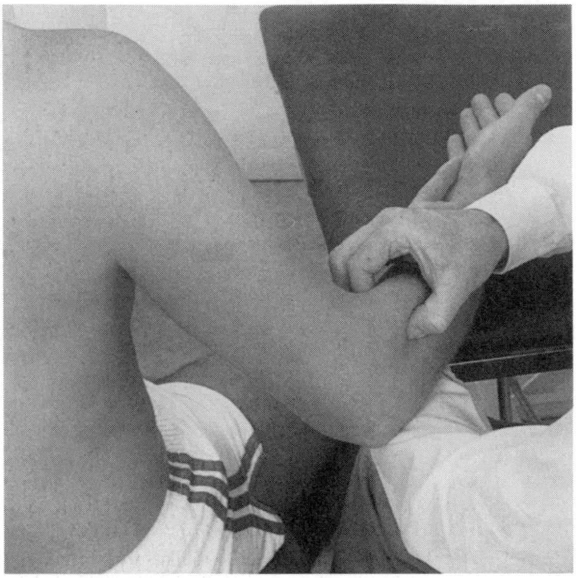

Palpation of the extensor carpi ulnaris muscle (Fig. 2.13)

The elbow and forearm are still held in the same starting position (90° flexion, supination). Place the palpating finger below the lateral epicondyle (A). Ask the subject to perform ulnar deviation of the wrist. Tension can be felt in the tendon of the extensor carpi ulnaris (Fig. 2.14 and Fig. 2.13, A), which runs towards the olecranon.

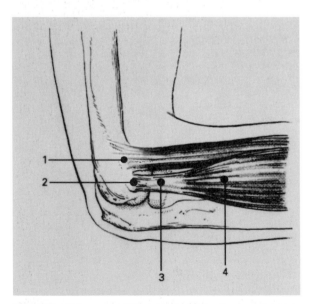

Fig. 2.11 Palpation of the muscle bellies of extensor carpi radialis longus and brevis.

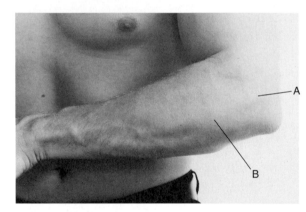

Fig. 2.13 View of the extensor carpi ulnaris muscle.

Fig. 2.12 Extensors of the wrist: 1, origin of extensor carpi radialis longus; 2, origin of extensor carpi radialis brevis; 3, tendon of extensor carpi radialis brevis; 4, belly of extensor carpi radialis brevis.

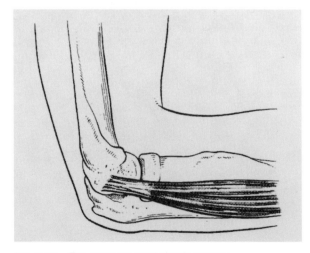

Fig. 2.14 The extensor carpi ulnaris muscle.

Palpation of the supinator muscle (Fig. 2.15)

Place the subject's elbow in 130–135° extension and in pronation. Identify the radius from the radial head downwards. Identify the ulna from the olecranon downwards. The supinator muscle (Fig. 2.16) is known to lie in the interspace between radius and ulna, between the elbow and mid-forearm. Ask the subject to supinate and resist this attempt. Contraction can be felt.

POSTERIOR

Bony landmarks (Figs 2.17 and 2.18)

Three bony prominences can be identified. On an extended elbow they lie in one line. Laterally is situated the lateral epicondyle (A) and medially the medial epicondyle (B). In between lies the olecranon (C), gross and prominent. During flexion of the elbow the olecranon moves downwards which makes its apex easily palpable. In a bent elbow the three bones form an isosceles triangle. Between the olecranon and the medial epicondyle lies the sulcus for the ulnar nerve (D).

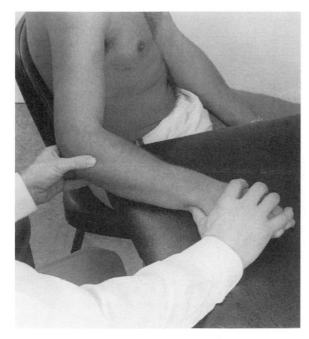

Fig. 2.15   Palpation of the supinator muscle.

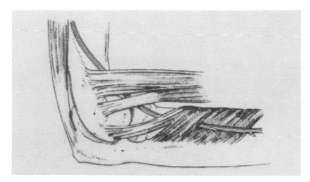

Fig. 2.16   The supinator muscle.

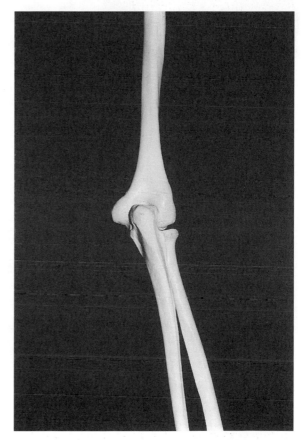

Fig. 2.17   Posterior view of the elbow (skeleton).

Palpation of soft tissue

(Figs 2.18 and 2.19)

Over the olecranon lies the olecranon bursa, which is only really palpable when it becomes inflamed and swollen.

Keep the subject's elbow flexed. Palpate for the upper border (apex) of the olecranon. Feel just lateral to this apex for the insertion of the tendon of the triceps muscle (E). Move the fingers upwards: a broad and flat tendon is felt and ends in the musculotendinous junction (F), shaped as an inverted U (Fig. 2.20).

Distally and slightly lateral to the olecranon the anconeus muscle (G) can be felt during an attempt to actively over-extend the elbow.

Palpation on a flexed elbow between the olecranon and the medial epicondyle discloses the sulcus in which the ulnar nerve – a soft and round structure – can be found. It is covered by the posterior part of the ulnar collateral ligament. The nerve courses under the medial head of the triceps muscle, then behind the medial epicondyle and then further distally in between the two heads of the flexor carpi ulnaris muscle, which form an aponeurotic arch.

The cubital tunnel

The cubital tunnel (Fig. 2.21) is built from the medial epicondyle, the olecranon, the ulnar collateral ligament and the aponeurotic arch.

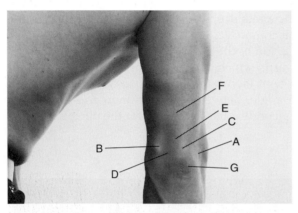

Fig. 2.18   Posterior view of the elbow (in vivo).

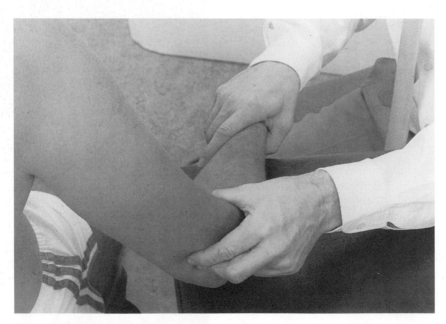

Fig. 2.19   Palpation of the triceps tendon.

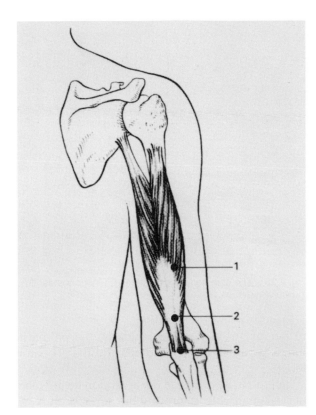

Fig. 2.20   The triceps muscle: 1, musculotendinous junction; 2, body of the tendon; 3, tenoperiosteal insertion.

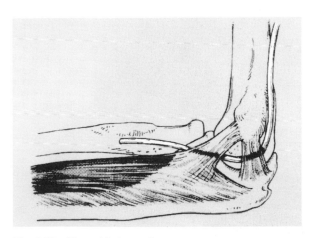

Fig. 2.21   The cubital tunnel.

MEDIAL

Bony landmarks (Fig. 2.22)

The medial epicondyle is recognized as a very prominent bone, which lies just subcutaneously.

Palpation of soft tissue
(Figs 2.23 and 2.24)

Keep the subject's elbow almost completely extended and in full supination. Move the finger from the medial aspect of the medial epicondyle (A) about 1–1.5 cm towards the anterior aspect. Palpate for a tough round structure. This is the common tendon of the flexors (Fig. 2.25 and Fig. 2.23, B).

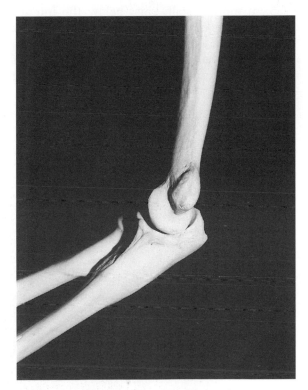

Fig. 2.22   Medial view of the elbow (skeleton).

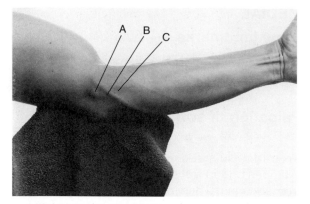

Fig. 2.23 Medial view of the elbow (in vivo).

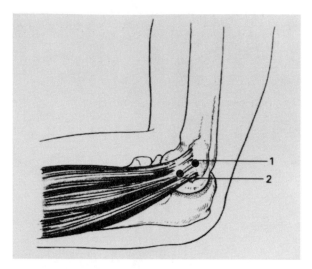

Fig. 2.25 The common flexor tendon: 1, tenoperiosteal; 2, musculotendinous.

0.5 cm more distally, just below the inferior border of the epicondyle and with the elbow slightly flexed, a thick and round muscular mass is palpable: the musculotendinous junction of this flexor group (C) consisting of, from medial to lateral: the flexor carpi ulnaris, the palmaris longus, the flexor carpi radialis and the pronator teres.

Lateral to the common flexor tendon the median nerve is palpable as a round but soft structure.

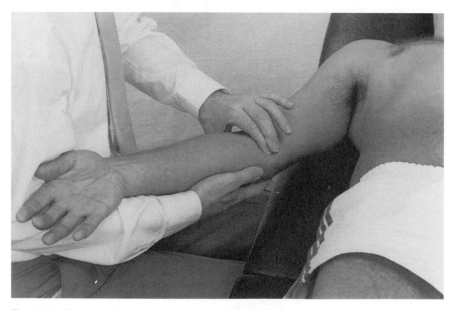

Fig. 2.24 Palpation of the common tendon of the flexors.

FUNCTIONAL EXAMINATION OF THE ELBOW

PASSIVE TESTS

Passive flexion

Positioning. The subject stands with the arm outstretched. The examiner stands level with the subject's arm. He places one hand against the back of the shoulder and grasps the distal forearm with the other hand.

Procedure. Bring the hand towards the shoulder, thereby stabilizing the latter, until the movement comes to a stop (Fig. 2.26).

Common mistakes. Inadequate stabilization allows the shoulder to move backwards.

Normal functional anatomy:
- *Range*: about 160°
- *End-feel*:
  - in well muscled subjects: a soft stop by tissue approximation, the muscles of the forearm coming in contact with the muscles of the upper arm
  - in poorly muscled subjects: a rather hard stop of bone engaging with bone.
- *Limiting structures*:
  - in well muscled subjects: the muscular masses of the upper arm and forearm coming in contact with each other
  - in poorly muscled subjects: bony contact between (1) the coronoid fossa of the humerus and coronoid process of the ulna and (2) the head of the radius and radial fossa of the humerus
  - tension in the posterior part of the joint capsule.

Common pathological situations:
- Painful limitation occurs in arthritis (as part of the capsular type of limitation) or when a loose body is present in the anterior part of the joint.
- Painless limitation is present in uncomplicated arthrosis.

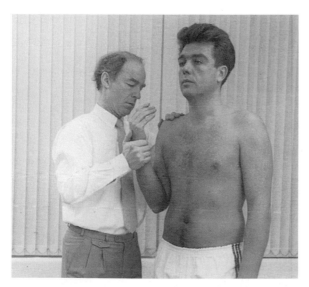

Fig. 2.26 Passive flexion.

Passive extension

Positioning. The subject stands with the arm outstretched. The examiner stands level with the subject's elbow. One hand stabilizes the elbow, and the other hand grasps the distal forearm.

Procedure:
- To test the range: move hands in opposite directions – distal hand downwards and proximal hand upwards (Fig. 2.27).
- To test the end-feel: bring the subject's elbow into slight flexion and move hands abruptly but gently in opposite directions towards extension.

Common mistakes. The elbow is not in complete supination.

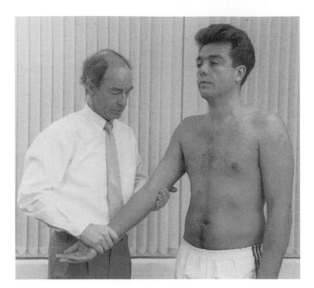

Fig. 2.27 Passive extension.

Normal functional anatomy:
- *Range*: generally 0° in the male; in female subjects and in hypermobile persons overextension of a few degrees may be possible
- *End-feel*: hard stop of bone engaging with bone
- *Limiting structures*:
  - bony contact between the olecranon process and olecranon fossa
  - tension in the anterior part of the joint capsule.

Common pathological situations:
- A painful limitation occurs in arthritis of the elbow joint and also when a loose body is present in the posterior part of the joint.
- A painless limitation is present in uncomplicated arthrosis.

Passive pronation

Positioning. The subject stands with the arm hanging and the elbow bent to a right angle. The examiner stands in front of the subject. Both hands encircle the distal forearm in such a way that the heel of the contralateral hand is placed against the volar part of the ulna and the fingers of the other hand against the dorsal aspect of the radius.

Procedure. Bring the subject's forearm into full pronation by a simultaneous movement of both hands in opposite directions (Fig. 2.28).

Common mistakes:
- The subject's shoulder is brought into abduction.
- Too much local pressure on the radius/ulna may provoke tenderness.

Normal functional anatomy:
- *Range*: about 85°
- *End-feel*: elastic
- *Limiting structures*: stretching of the interosseous membrane and squeezing of the insertion of the bicipital tendon between the radial tuberosity and the ulna.

Common pathological situations. The movement is painful in lesions of the proximal radioulnar joint, in bicipitoradial bursitis and in tendinitis of the biceps brachii at the insertion onto the radial tuberosity.

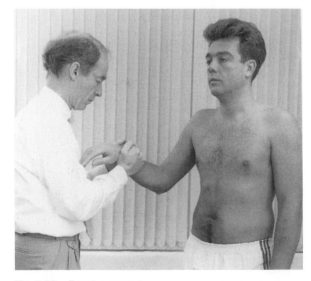

Fig. 2.28 Passive pronation.

Passive supination

Positioning. The subject stands with the arm hanging and the elbow bent to a right angle. The examiner stands in front of the subject. Both hands encircle the distal forearm in such a way that the heel of the ipsilateral hand is placed against the dorsal part of the ulna and the fingers of the other hand against the volar aspect of the radius.

Procedure. Bring the subject's forearm into full supination by a simultaneous movement of both hands in opposite directions (Fig. 2.29).

Common mistakes. Too much local pressure on the radius/ulna may provoke tenderness.

Normal functional anatomy:
- *Range*: about 90°
- *End-feel*: elastic
- *Limiting structures*:
  - tension in the interosseous membrane, the oblique cord and the anterior ligament of the distal radioulnar joint
  - tension in the extensor carpi ulnaris tendon when the posterior aspect of the ulnar

notch of the radius impacts against the styloid process of the ulna.

Common pathological situations. The movement is painful when the proximal radioulnar joint is affected.

ISOMETRIC CONTRACTIONS
Resisted flexion

Positioning. The subject stands with the arm hanging, the elbow flexed to a right angle and the forearm supinated. The examiner stands level with the elbow. One hand is on the distal part of the forearm and the other hand on top of the shoulder.

Procedure. Resist the subject's attempt to flex the elbow (Fig. 2.30).

Common mistakes:
- In strong subjects flexion cannot sufficiently be resisted if the resistance is not given perpendicular to the subject's forearm.
- Movement is allowed at the elbow.
- The subject performs shoulder elevation.

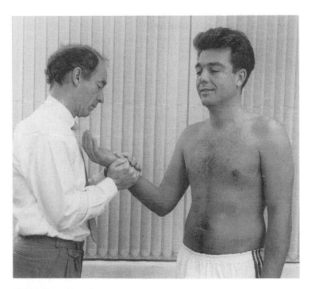

Fig. 2.29   Passive supination.

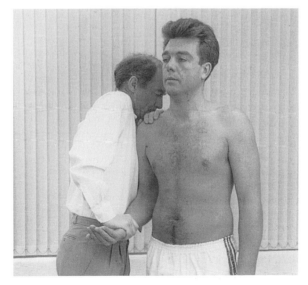

Fig. 2.30   Resisted flexion.

Anatomical structures tested:

Muscle function:
* *Important flexors*:
  – Brachialis
  – Biceps brachii
* *Less important flexors*:
  – Brachioradialis
  – Extensor carpi radialis longus
  – Pronator teres.

Neural function:

Muscle	Innervation	
	Peripheral	Nerve root
Brachialis	Musculocutaneous	C5–C6
Biceps brachii	Musculocutaneous	C5–C6
Brachioradialis	Radial	C5–C6
Extensor carpi radialis longus	Radial	C6–C7
Pronator teres	Median	C6–C7

Common pathological situations:
* Pain indicates a lesion of either the biceps brachii or the brachialis muscle.
* Painless weakness occurs in either a C5 or a C6 nerve root lesion.
* Painful weakness is suggestive of an avulsion fracture of the radial tuberosity.

Resisted extension

Positioning. The subject stands with the arm alongside the body, the elbow flexed to 90° and the forearm in supination. The examiner stands level with the elbow. One hand supports the distal part of the forearm and the other hand is on top of the shoulder.

Procedure. Resist the subject's attempt to extend the elbow (Fig. 2.31).

Common mistakes:
* In strong subjects, flexion cannot sufficiently be resisted if the resistance is not given perpendicular to the subject's forearm.
* Movement is allowed at the elbow.

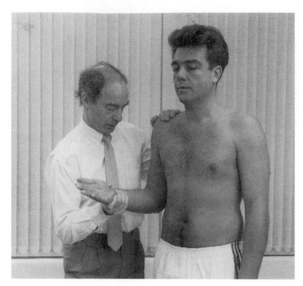

Fig. 2.31   Resisted extension.

Anatomical structures tested:

Muscle function:
* *Most important extensor*:
  – Triceps brachii
* *Less important extensor*:
  – Anconeus.

Neural function:

Muscle	Innervation	
	Peripheral	Nerve root
Triceps brachii	Radial	C7–C8
Anconeus	Radial	C7–C8

Common pathological situations:
* The test is painful when a lesion of the triceps is present.
* Weakness occurs in lesions of either the radial nerve or the C7 nerve root.
* Painful weakness may indicate a partial rupture of the triceps or a fracture of the olecranon.

Resisted pronation

Positioning. The subject stands with the arm alongside the body, the elbow bent to a right angle and the forearm in neutral position. The examiner stands in front of the subject. The ipsilateral hand carries the forearm, the thenar against the palmar and distal aspect of the radius and the fingers against the dorsal aspect of the ulna. The other hand reinforces: thenar on ulna and fingers on radius.

Procedure. Resist the subject's attempt to pronate the forearm (Fig. 2.32).

Common mistakes:
- The subject abducts the shoulder.
- Too much local pressure on the radius/ulna may provoke tenderness.
- Movement is allowed at the elbow.

Anatomical structures tested:

Muscle function:
- Pronator teres
- Pronator quadratus.

Neural function:

Muscle	Innervation	
	Peripheral	Nerve root
Pronator teres	Median	C6–C7
Pronator quadratus	Median	C8–T1

Common pathological situations. Pain occurs in golfer's elbow – a lesion of the common flexor tendon – or in an isolated lesion of the pronator teres muscle.

Resisted supination

Positioning. The subject stands with the arm alongside the body, the elbow bent to 90° and the forearm in neutral position. The examiner stands in front of the subject. The ipsilateral hand carries the forearm, the thenar against the distal and palmar aspect of the ulna. The thenar of the other hand is placed against the dorsal aspect of the radius.

Procedure. Resist the subject's attempt to supinate the forearm (Fig. 2.33).

Common mistakes:
- The subject extends the elbow.
- Movement is allowed at the elbow.
- Too much local pressure on the radius/ulna may provoke tenderness.

Anatomical structures tested:

Muscle function:
- *Most important supinators*:
  - Supinator
  - Biceps brachii

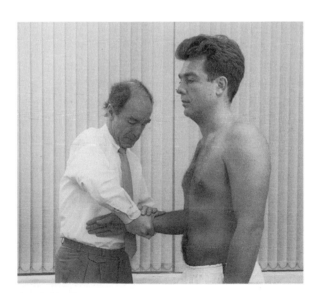

Fig. 2.32 Resisted pronation.

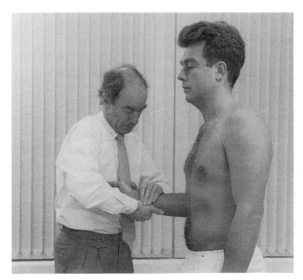

Fig. 2.33 Resisted supination.

- *Less important supinator*:
  - Brachioradialis.

Neural function:

Muscle	Innervation	
	Peripheral	Nerve root
Supinator	Radial	C5–C6
Biceps brachii	Musculocutaneous	C5–C6
Brachioradialis	Radial	C5–C8

Common pathological situations. Pain is the result of a lesion of the biceps or, more rarely, a lesion of the supinator muscle.

Resisted extension of the wrist

Positioning. The subject stands with the arm hanging, the elbow extended and the wrist in neutral position (between pronation and supination, and between flexion and extension). The examiner stands level with the subject's elbow. The contralateral arm lifts and carries the elbow and keeps it extended. The hand stabilizes the forearm. The other hand is placed at the dorsum of the subject's hand.

Procedure. Resist the subject's attempt to extend the wrist (Fig. 2.34).

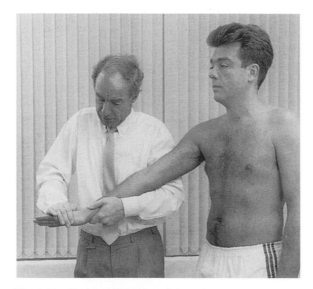

Fig. 2.34 Resisted extension of the wrist.

Common mistakes:
- The subject is allowed to lift the arm up.
- The elbow is allowed to flex. This can be prevented by the examiner's arm keeping the subject's elbow well raised.
- The wrist is not held in neutral position, which puts stress on non-contractile structures.

Anatomical structures tested:

Muscle function:
- *Important wrist extensors*:
  - Extensor digitorum communis
  - Extensor carpi radialis longus
  - Extensor carpi radialis brevis
  - Extensor carpi ulnaris
- *Less important wrist extensors*:
  - Extensor indicis proprius
  - Extensor pollicis longus
  - Extensor digiti minimi.

Neural function:

Muscle	Innervation	
	Peripheral	Nerve root
Extensor digitorum communis	Radial	C6–C8
Extensor carpi radialis longus	Radial	C6–C7
Extensor carpi radialis brevis	Radial	C7
Extensor carpi ulnaris	Radial	C7–C8
Extensor indicis proprius	Radial	C6–C8
Extensor pollicis longus	Radial	C7–C8
Extensor digiti minimi	Radial	C6–C8

Common pathological situations:
- When elbow pain is elicited, tennis elbow – a lesion in the radial extensors of the wrist – is most probable. Other possibilities are a lesion of the extensor carpi ulnaris or of the extensor digitorum.
- Weakness may result from a radial nerve lesion or from either the C6 or C8 nerve root. Bilateral weakness suggests either lead poisoning, or bronchus carcinoma, or a more general neurological disease.

Resisted flexion of the wrist

Positioning. The subject stands with the arm hanging, the elbow extended and the wrist in neutral position (between pronation and supination, and between flexion and extension). The examiner stands level with the subject's elbow. The contralateral arm lifts and carries the elbow and keeps it extended. The hand stabilizes the forearm. The other hand is placed at the palm of the subject's hand.

Procedure. Resist the subject's attempt to flex the wrist (Fig. 2.35).

Common mistakes:
- The subject is allowed to push the arm down.

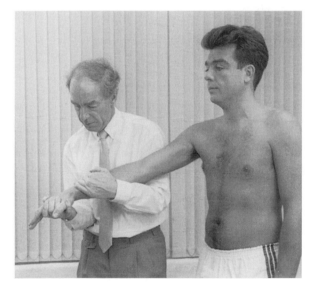

Fig. 2.35   Resisted flexion of the wrist.

If this happens it is the result of inadequate fixation.
- The wrist is not held in neutral position, which puts stress on non-contractile structures.

Anatomical structures tested:

Muscle function:
- *Important wrist flexors*:
  - Flexor digitorum superficialis
  - Flexor digitorum profundus
  - Flexor carpi ulnaris
  - Flexor carpi radialis
- *Less important wrist flexors*:
  - Abductor pollicis longus
  - Palmaris longus.

Neural function:

Muscle	Innervation	
	Peripheral	Nerve root
Flexor digitorum superficialis	Median	C7–T1
Flexor digitorum profundus	Median	C7–T1
Flexor carpi ulnaris	Ulnar	C7–C8
Flexor carpi radialis	Median	C7–T1
Abductor pollicis longus	Radial	C7–C8
Palmaris longus	Median	C7–T1

Common pathological situations:
- Pain at the elbow occurs in golfer's elbow – a lesion in the common flexor tendon.
- Weakness suggests a C7 or C8 nerve root lesion.

3

Wrist

SURFACE AND PALPATORY ANATOMY

RADIAL

Bony landmarks (Figs 3.1, 3.2 and 3.3)

At the distal end of the radius the styloid process (A) can be palpated. Slightly more proximally on the radius a small groove can be found. Just distally to the styloid process the scaphoid (navicular) bone (B) is palpable. It can be made more prominent by asking the subject to execute ulnar deviation of the wrist. When the palpating finger is on the navicular bone it lies in a depression between two tendons, called the 'anatomical snuffbox'. At the distal end of the snuffbox the joint line can be palpated between the scaphoid bone and the trapezium, especially

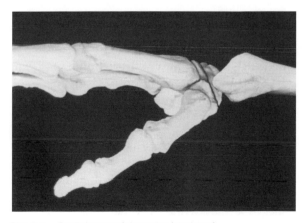

Fig. 3.1   Radial view of the wrist (skeleton).

39

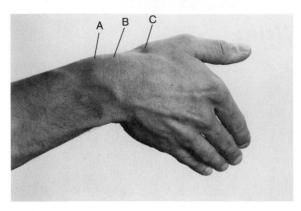

Fig. 3.2 Bony landmarks at the radial side of the wrist (in vivo).

Palpation of soft tissue

Place the palpating finger just distally to the styloid process and feel for the tightening of the radial collateral ligament during ulnar deviation. It attaches to the scaphoid bone (Fig. 3.4).

Move the finger slightly towards the palmar aspect. Ask the subject to extend the thumb (Fig. 3.5). Two strong tendons can be recognized (Fig. 3.6): first the extensor pollicis brevis (A), which is seen to run towards the base of the proximal phalanx. It forms the radial border of the 'anatomical snuffbox'. Next to it the abductor

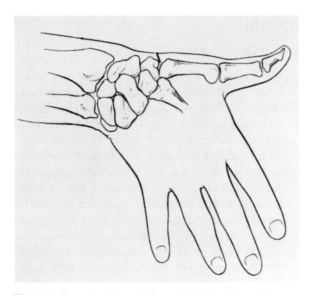

Fig. 3.3 Bony structures at the radial side of the wrist.

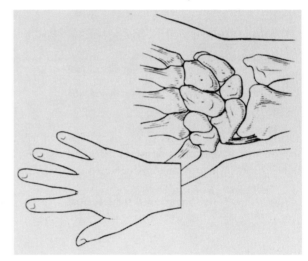

Fig. 3.4 The radial collateral ligament.

when the subject moves the thumb. 6–7 mm more distally another joint line is palpable – the one between the trapezium bone and the first metacarpal bone. This joint line is well palpable during movement of the first metacarpal bone: feel for the shaft of the first metacarpal bone with one finger and move proximally towards the base of the bone (C). The joint line can be felt just proximally to the proximal border of the bone, especially while the other hand moves the first metacarpal to and fro.

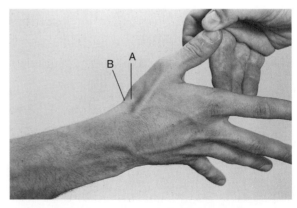

Fig. 3.5 View of the extensors and abductor of the thumb.

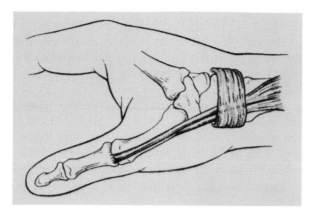

Fig. 3.6 Tendons at the radial aspect of the wrist.

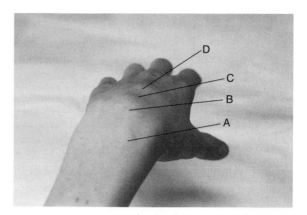

Fig. 3.8 Bony landmarks at the dorsal side of the wrist (in vivo).

pollicis longus (B) is felt, inserting at the base of the first metacarpal bone.

DORSAL

Bony landmarks (Figs 3.7 and 3.8)

Radius and ulna are easily palpable. The styloid process of the radius descends a bit further distally than the styloid process of the ulna.

The distal radioulnar joint can be recognized by grasping the distal end of the radius with one hand and the distal end of the ulna with the other, and by moving both hands in opposite directions.

The distal border of the radius is sharp and can be felt as being the proximal border of the

radiocarpal joint, which has a wide joint line. One finger-width more proximally, on the dorsal aspect of the radius, a nodular bone can be felt. This is the dorsal tubercle (A) of the radius which forms an important landmark. At the ulnar side the thick head of the ulna is palpated.

The carpal bones consist of two rows. In the proximal row lie the scaphoid, lunate, triquetral and pisiform bones.

Distal to the inferior border of the radius, two bones can be palpated. The most radial one is the already detected scaphoid bone. It is felt more clearly during ulnar deviation of the wrist. The most ulnar bone is the lunate bone (B), which is palpable on a flexed wrist. Ulnar to the lunate and articulating with the ulna lies the triquetral bone. It is felt to move when the hand is again brought into radial deviation.

The distal row contains the trapezium, trapezoid, capitate and hamate bones.

Distal and a bit more radially to the scaphoid lies the trapezium. Between the lunate and the base of the third metacarpal bone a depression (C) is felt in which the capitate bone is palpable. The capitate articulates with the base of the third metacarpal bone (D). The bone between the capitate and the trapezium is the trapezoid bone, which is more difficult to palpate.

To the ulnar side of the capitate and somewhat more distal and radial than the triquetral, the hamate bone is felt; it articulates mainly with the fourth metacarpal bone.

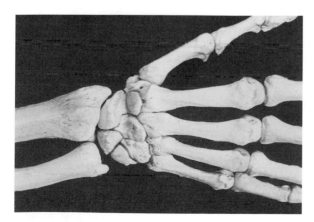

Fig. 3.7 Dorsal view of the wrist (skeleton).

Palpation of soft tissue

Place one finger just radially to the dorsal tubercle of the radius (A) (Fig. 3.9). Ask the subject to make a first and to squeeze and unsqueeze it. During this action tendinous tightening can be felt. These are the tendons of the extensor carpi radialis longus and extensor carpi radialis brevis (Fig. 3.10). When the subject continues these muscular contractions the tendons can be followed, approximately 2 cm more distally, until the point where they separate (B). The most radial tendon (longus) (C) is felt to insert at the radial aspect of the base of the second metacarpal bone and the more ulnar tendon (brevis) (D) inserts at the radial aspect of the base of the third metacarpal bone (Fig. 3.11).

Place one finger just ulnar to the dorsal tubercle of the radius. Ask the subject to extend the thumb. Feel for the extensor pollicis longus (Fig. 3.12, A) tendon, which is the ulnar border of the anatomical snuffbox. It can be palpated until its insertion onto the distal phalanx of the

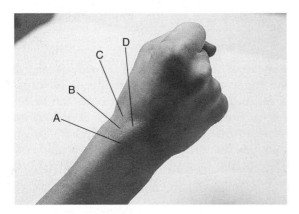

Fig. 3.9   View of the extensors of the wrist (in vivo).

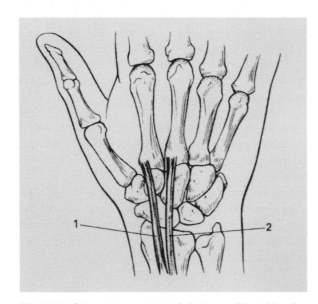

Fig. 3.10   The extensor carpi radialis longus (1) and brevis (2).

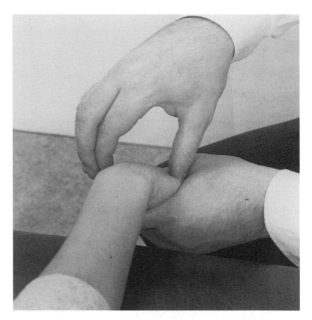

Fig. 3.11   Palpation of the extensor carpi radialis longus.

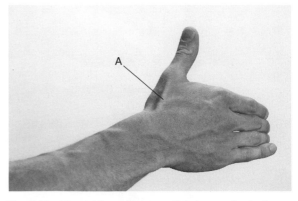

Fig. 3.12   View of the extensor pollicis longus (in vivo).

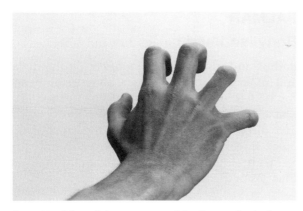

Fig. 3.13 View of the extensors of the fingers (in vivo).

thumb: the tendon turns 45° around the dorsal tubercle of the radius, crosses over the extensor carpi radialis longus and brevis, and goes towards the thumb.

Palpate the dorsal aspect of the wrist while the subject extends the fingers. Movement can be felt of the tendons of the extensor digitorum communis and of the extensor indicis proprius. When one finger is extended at a time the different tendons can be palpated one by one.

Place one finger just radially to the head of the ulna. Ask the subject to extend the little finger and feel for the extensor digiti minimi. This tendon overlies the distal radioulnar joint.

Place one finger at the inferior and ulnar border of the head of the ulna (Fig. 3.14, A). Ask the subject to perform an ulnar deviation during extension. The strong and thick tendon of the

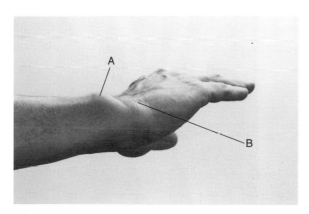

Fig. 3.14 View of the extensor carpi ulnaris (in vivo).

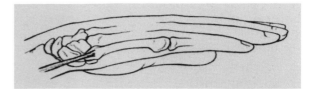

Fig. 3.15 The extensor carpi ulnaris.

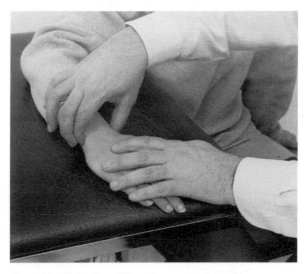

Fig. 3.16 Palpation of the extensor carpi ulnaris.

extensor carpi ulnaris (B) is felt (Figs 3.15 and 3.16). It can be followed to its insertion at the base of the fifth metacarpal bone.

ULNAR
Bony landmarks (Fig. 3.17)

At the distal end of the ulna the small styloid process (A) is palpable. Just distal to it the triquetral bone (B) becomes prominent when the subject moves the hand in radial deviation. When the palpating finger is moved even more distally and the hand is brought back to the neutral position the base of the fifth metacarpal bone (C) is encountered.

Palpation of soft tissue

Place the finger just distal to the styloid process and move the subject's hand in radial deviation.

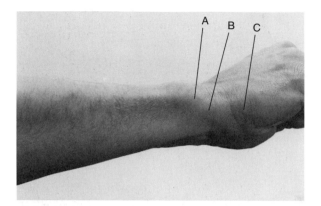

Fig. 3.17 Bony landmarks at the ulnar side of the wrist (in vivo).

Tightening can be felt of the ulnar collateral ligament (Fig. 3.18), which goes towards the triquetral bone. Ask the subject to move the hand towards the ulnar side and to extend the wrist slightly. Along the distal part of the ulna the tendon of the extensor carpi ulnaris is palpable.

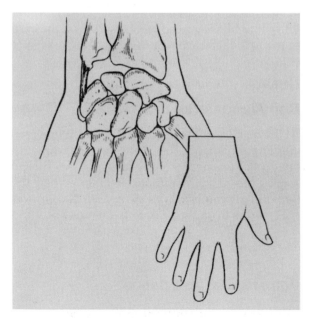

Fig. 3.18 The ulnar collateral ligament.

PALMAR
Bony landmarks (Figs 3.19 and 3.20)

Radius and ulna can be identified. At the distal and ulnar side of the ulna a bony prominence can be felt: the pisiform bone (A). Put the interphalangeal joint of the thumb onto the pisiform and direct the thumb towards the base of the index finger of the subject. Flex the thumb and feel its tip touch the hook of hamate through the muscles of the hypothenar.

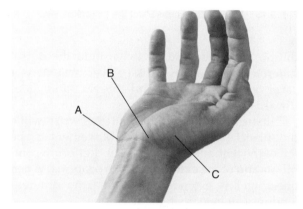

Fig. 3.19 Bony landmarks at the palmar side of the wrist (in vivo).

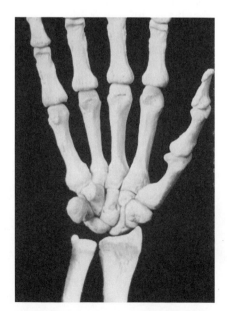

Fig. 3.20 Palmar view of the wrist (skeleton).

At the distal end of the radius the prominent tubercle of scaphoid (B) is well palpable. Put the interphalangeal joint of the thumb onto the scaphoid's tubercle and direct the thumb towards the base of the thumb. Flex the thumb and feel its tip touch the trapezium bone. Laterally and distal to it lies the base of the first metacarpal (C). When the finger moves from the scaphoid in the direction of the index finger, the base of the second metacarpal bone can be palpated through the muscles of the thenar.

The carpal tunnel (Figs 3.21, 3.22 and 3.23)

The carpal tunnel lies between – on the ulnar side – the pisiform bone (A) and the hook of the hamate bone (B) and – on the radial side – the tubercle of the scaphoid bone (C) and the trapezium bone (D).

It can be localized on the heel of the hand and somewhat towards the ulnar side. It is covered by the transverse ligament.

The content of the carpal tunnel is:

- the median nerve
- the flexor pollicis longus
- the flexor carpi radialis
- the flexor digitorum superficialis and profundus.

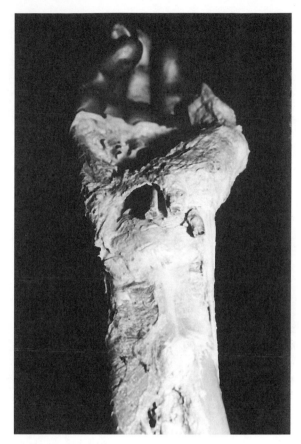

Fig. 3.22 View in the carpal tunnel (specimen).

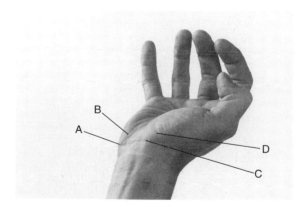

Fig. 3.21 Bony boundaries of the carpal tunnel (in vivo).

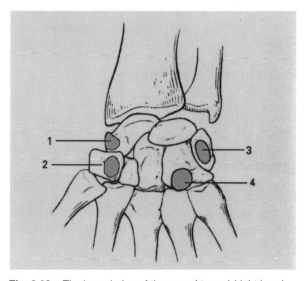

Fig. 3.23 The boundaries of the carpal tunnel (right hand, palmar view): 1, scaphoid; 2, trapezium; 3, pisiform; 4, hamate.

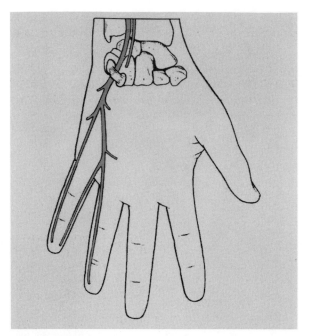

Fig. 3.24 The ulnar nerve passes through the tunnel of Guyon.

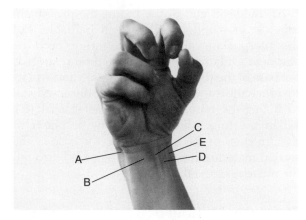

Fig. 3.25 View of the flexors of wrist and fingers (in vivo).

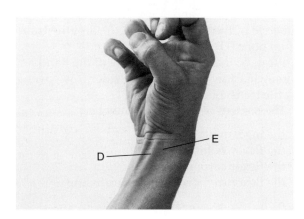

Fig. 3.26 Radial view of the wrist (in vivo).

The tunnel of Guyon (Fig. 3.24)

Palpate for the interspace between the pisiform and the hook of hamate. This is Guyon's tunnel that contains the ulnar nerve and ulnar artery and is covered by the pisohamate ligament.

Palpation of soft tissue
(Figs 3.25 and 3.26)

Feel for the pisiform bone and place the palpating finger against its proximal aspect. Ask the subject to actively abduct the little finger. The tightening of the flexor carpi ulnaris (A) can be felt (Figs 3.27 and 3.28). The tendon can now be followed distal to the pisiform until its insertion on the base of the fifth metacarpal bone. The pisiform is a sesamoid bone in the tendon of the flexor carpi ulnaris.

Place the thumb radial to the previous tendon at the distal part of the forearm. It now lies on the tendons of the flexor digitorum superficialis (B),

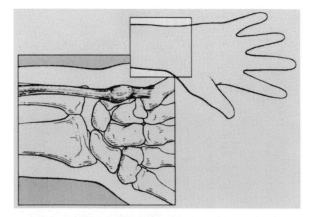

Fig. 3.27 The flexor carpi ulnaris.

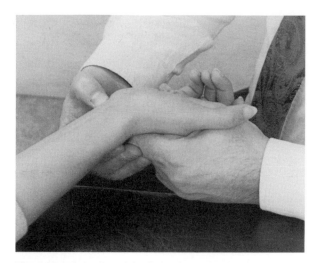

Fig. 3.28 Palpation of the flexor carpi ulnaris.

of which the movement can be felt during active flexion and extension of the fingers (Fig. 3.29).

In a deeper layer the presence of the flexor digitorum profundus can be imagined.

Move the finger a bit more towards the radial side and ask the subject to oppose the thumb and little finger and to simultaneously flex the wrist. The thin tendon of the palmaris longus (C)

becomes prominent. It inserts into the palmar aponeurosis of the hand. (It has to be remembered that this muscle is inconstant.)

Approximately 1 cm radially to the palmaris longus the strong and thick tendon of the flexor carpi radialis (D) is palpable (Fig. 3.30), especially when the subject flexes and radially deviates the wrist. It inserts at the base of the second metacarpal bone (Fig. 3.31).

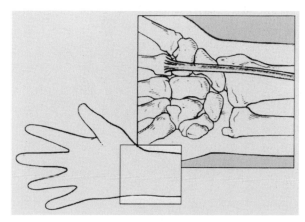

Fig. 3.30 The flexor carpi radialis.

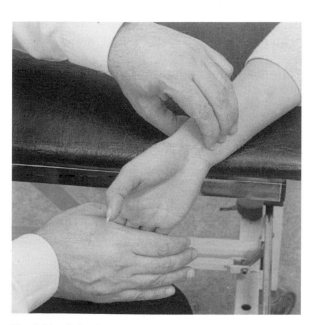

Fig. 3.29 Palpation of the flexor digitorum superficialis.

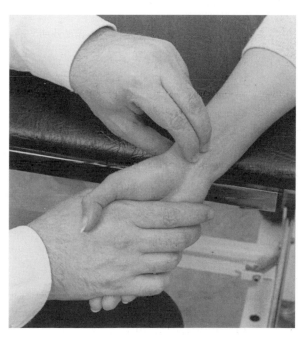

Fig. 3.31 Palpation of the flexor carpi radialis.

In between the palmaris longus and the flexor carpi radialis, in a deeper layer, the tendon of the flexor pollicis longus can be felt to move during flexion and extension movements of the thumb (Figs 3.32 and 3.33).

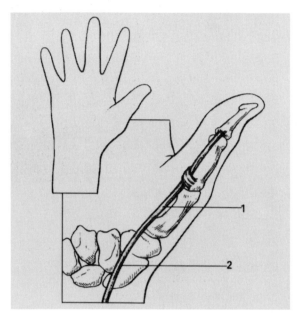

Fig. 3.32 The flexor pollicis longus: 1, level of the first metacarpal; 2, level of the carpus.

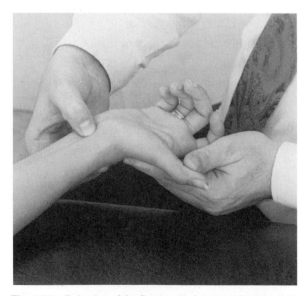

Fig. 3.33 Palpation of the flexor pollicis longus (at the wrist).

Between the flexor carpi radialis and the abductor pollicis longus the pulsations of the radial artery (E) can be felt.

FUNCTIONAL EXAMINATION OF THE WRIST

Introduction/general remarks

Examination of the wrist should include all structures that can be responsible for pain felt in the region called 'wrist' by the patient.

This comprises the distal radioulnar joint, the wrist joint, the trapezium–first metacarpal joint and also the tendons that control the wrist, thumb and fingers and the intrinsic muscles of the hand.

PASSIVE TESTS OF THE DISTAL RADIOULNAR JOINT

Passive pronation

Positioning. The subject stands with the arm hanging and the elbow bent to 90°. The examiner stands in front of the subject. Both hands encircle the distal part of the forearm in such a way that the heel of the contralateral hand is placed on the palmar aspect of the ulna and the fingers of the other hand lie at the dorsal aspect of the radius.

Procedure. Bring the subject's forearm into full pronation by a simultaneous action of both hands in opposite directions (Fig. 3.34).

Common mistakes:
- The subject is allowed to abduct the shoulder.
- Too much pressure on the radius or ulna may provoke local tenderness.

Normal functional anatomy:
- *Range*: about 85°
- *End-feel*: elastic
- *Limiting structures*: impaction of the radius against the ulna together with stretching of the interosseous membrane.

Common pathological situations. Pain at full

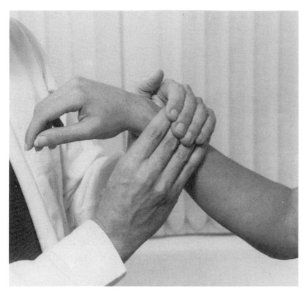

Fig. 3.34 Passive pronation.

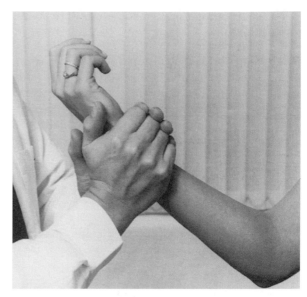

Fig. 3.35 Passive supination.

range suggests arthritis or arthrosis of the distal radioulnar joint.

Passive supination

Positioning. The subject stands with the arm hanging and the elbow bent to 90°. The examiner stands in front of the subject. Both hands encircle the distal part of the forearm in such a way that the heel of the ipsilateral hand is placed on the dorsal aspect of the ulna and the fingers of the other hand at the palmar aspect of the radius.

Procedure. Bring the subject's forearm into full supination by a simultaneous movement of both hands in opposite directions (Fig. 3.35).

Common mistakes. Too much pressure on radius or ulna may provoke local tenderness.

Normal functional anatomy:
- *Range*: about 90°
- *End-feel*: elastic
- *Limiting structures*:
  - tension in the interosseous membrane, the oblique cord and the anterior ligament of the distal radioulnar joint

- tension in the extensor carpi ulnaris tendon when the posterior aspect of the ulnar notch of the radius impacts against the styloid process of the ulna.

Common pathological situations:
- Pain at full range occurs in arthritis or arthrosis of the distal radioulnar joint and also in tendinitis of the extensor carpi ulnaris level with the distal end of the ulna.
- Limitation indicates a malunited Colles' fracture.

PASSIVE TESTS OF THE WRIST JOINT

Remark

The wrist joint has a proximal part – the radiocarpal joint – and a distal one – the intercarpal joint. The tests described in this chapter test the wrist joint as a whole and do not test its structures separately.

All movements are executed with the wrist held in the neutral position:

- halfway between flexion and extension
- halfway between radial and ulnar deviation.

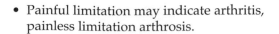

The positioning for all passive tests of the wrist joint is the same.

Positioning for testing the mobility of the wrist. The subject stands with the arm hanging, the elbow flexed to a right angle and the forearm pronated. The examiner stands next to the subject. The contralateral hand carries the subject's forearm, which is kept between the examiner's arm and trunk. The other hand grasps the subject's hand distally on the metacarpals.

Passive flexion

Procedure. Bring the subject's wrist into maximal flexion (Fig. 3.36).

Common mistakes. None.

Normal functional anatomy:
- *Range*: 85°
- *End-feel*: Elastic
- *Limiting structures*: stretching of the dorsal ligaments of the carpus, of the intercarpal ligaments and the capsules of the different intercarpal joints.

Common pathological situations:
- Pain at the dorsal aspect occurs in a lesion of the dorsal ligaments or the extensor tendons of the wrist.
- Pain at the palmar aspect may occur in periostitis, mostly of the scaphoid bone.

- Painful limitation may indicate arthritis, painless limitation arthrosis.

Passive extension

Procedure. Bring the subject's wrist into maximal extension (Fig. 3.37).

Common mistakes. None.

Normal functional anatomy:
- *Range*: 85°
- *End-feel*: rather hard
- *Limiting structures*:
  - stretching of the palmar ligaments of the carpus and of the intercarpal ligaments and capsules
  - contact of the proximal row of carpal bones against the radius.

Common pathological situations:
- Pain at full range and felt at the dorsal aspect may suggest a periostitis of the distal epiphysis of the radius or a dorsal ganglion. Palmar pain may be provoked in a lesion of the palmar ligament of the wrist or of one of the flexor tendons.
- Painful limitation is present in arthritis, carpal subluxation – usually of the capitate bone – and aseptic necrosis, usually of the lunate bone.
- Painless limitation is typical for arthrosis.

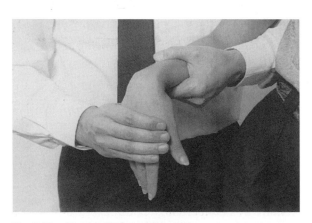

Fig. 3.36 Passive flexion of the wrist.

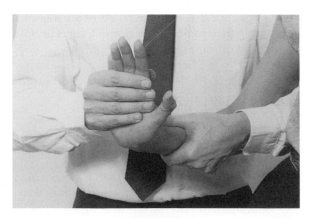

Fig. 3.37 Passive extension of the wrist.

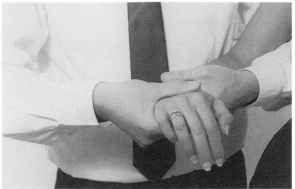

Fig. 3.38   Passive radial deviation of the wrist.

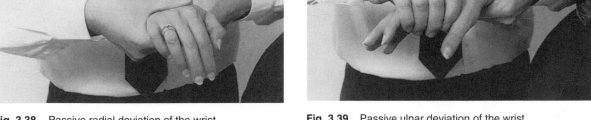

Fig. 3.39   Passive ulnar deviation of the wrist.

Passive radial deviation

Procedure. Push the subject's wrist to the radial side until the end of range is reached (Fig. 3.38).

Common mistakes. None.

Normal functional anatomy:
* *Range*: about 15°
* *End-feel*: rather hard
* *Limiting structures*: stretching of the ulnar collateral ligament and of the extensor carpi ulnaris.

Common pathological situations:
* Pain at the ulnar side is typical for a lesion of the ulnar collateral ligament or the extensor carpi ulnaris.
* Pain at the radial side may be provoked in de Quervain's disease as the result of gliding of the tendons of abductor pollicis longus and extensor pollicis brevis in their inflamed sheath.

Passive ulnar deviation

Procedure. Pull the subject's wrist to the ulnar side until the end of range is reached (Fig. 3.39).

Common mistakes. The thumb is included in the movement: it should be left free to avoid excessive stretching of the tendons of the extensors and long abductor.

Normal functional anatomy:
* *Range*: about 45°
* *End-feel*: rather hard
* *Limiting structures*: radial collateral ligament.

Common pathological situations:
* Pain at the radial side at full range is present in a sprain of the radial collateral ligament or as the result of gliding of tendons in an inflamed sheath in tenovaginitis of abductor pollicis longus and extensor pollicis brevis (de Quervain's disease).
* Pain at the ulnar side can be elicited by a lesion of the triangular fibrocartilaginous complex.

PASSIVE TEST FOR THE TRAPEZIUM–FIRST METACARPAL JOINT
Backwards movement during extension

Positioning. The subject stands with the arm hanging and the elbow bent to 90° and in supination. The examiner faces the subject. One hand grasps the hand and stabilizes it.

Procedure. The other hand moves the thumb into extension first and then backwards (Fig. 3.40).

Common mistakes. The thumb is hyperextended in the metacarpophalangeal joint, so that most

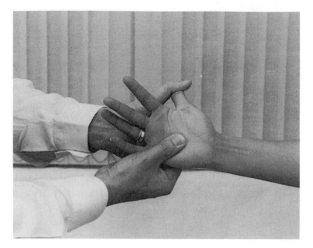

Fig. 3.40 Passive movement of the thumb.

stress falls on this joint and not on the trapezium–first metacarpal one.

Normal functional anatomy:
- *Range*: until the movement stops
- *End-feel*: elastic
- *Limiting structures*: stretching of the anterolateral part of the joint capsule of the trapezium–first metacarpal joint.

Common pathological situations:
- Pain indicates arthritis or arthrosis ('rhizarthrosis') generally of the joint between the trapezium and the first metacarpal bones. More exceptionally it is the joint between trapezium and scaphoid bones.
- Excessive range of motion occurs after rupture of the ulnar aspect of the metacarpophalangeal joint capsule.

ISOMETRIC CONTRACTIONS
Muscles controlling the wrist

Remarks

As most muscles take their origin at the elbow and overrun it, the subject's elbow should always be held in extension to put maximal stress on these structures.

All movements are executed with the wrist held in the neutral position:
- halfway between flexion and extension
- halfway between radial and ulnar deviation. The positioning is the same for the four tests.

Positioning for testing the resisted movements of the wrist. The subject stands with the arm hanging, the elbow extended and the forearm in neutral position. The examiner stands level with the subject's elbow. The contralateral arm lifts and carries the elbow and keeps it extended. The hand stabilizes the forearm. The other hand grasps the subject's hand distally on the metacarpals to apply resistance.

Resisted flexion

Procedure. Resist the subject's attempt to flex the wrist (Fig. 3.41).

Common mistakes:
- The subject is allowed to push the arm down. If this happens it is the result of inadequate fixation.
- The elbow is not held in extension.

Anatomical structures tested:

Muscle function:
- *Important wrist flexors*:
  - Flexor digitorum superficialis

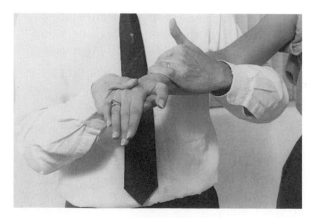

Fig. 3.41 Resisted flexion of the wrist.

- Flexor digitorum profundus
- Flexor carpi ulnaris
- Flexor carpi radialis
• *Less important wrist flexors*:
    - Abductor pollicis longus
    - Palmaris longus.

Neural function:

Muscle	Innervation	
	Peripheral	Nerve root
Flexor digitorum superficialis	Median	C7–T1
Flexor digitorum profundus	Median	C7–T1
Flexor carpi ulnaris	Ulnar	C7–C8
Flexor carpi radialis	Median	C7–T1
Abductor pollicis longus	Radial	C7–C8
Palmaris longus	Median	C7–T1

Common pathological situations:
• Pain at the wrist occurs in tendinitis of the flexor carpi radialis, flexor carpi ulnaris and flexor digitorum profundus.
• Weakness is found in C7 and C8 nerve root lesions.

Resisted extension

Procedure. Resist the subject's attempt to extend the wrist (Fig. 3.42).

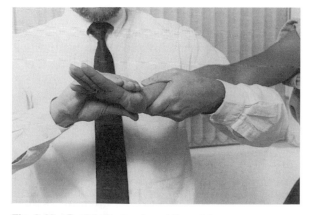

Fig. 3.42 Resisted extension of the wrist.

Common mistakes:
• The subject is allowed to push the arm upwards. If this happens it is the result of inadequate fixation.
• The elbow is not held in extension.

Anatomical structures tested:

Muscle function:
• *Important wrist extensors*:
    - Extensor digitorum communis
    - Extensor carpi radialis longus
    - Extensor carpi radialis brevis
    - Extensor carpi ulnaris
• *Less important wrist extensors*:
    - Extensor indicis proprius
    - Extensor pollicis longus
    - Extensor digiti minimi.

Neural function:

Muscle	Innervation	
	Peripheral	Nerve root
Extensor digitorum communis	Radial	C6–C8
Extensor carpi radialis longus	Radial	C6–C7
Extensor carpi radialis brevis	Radial	C7
Extensor carpi ulnaris	Radial	C7–C8
Extensor indicis proprius	Radial	C6–C8
Extensor pollicis longus	Radial	C7–C8
Extensor digiti minimi	Radial	C6–C8

Common pathological situations:
• Pain at the wrist is indicative of tendinitis of extensor carpi radialis longus and/or brevis, extensor carpi ulnaris, extensor indicis proprius or extensor digitorum communis.
• Unilateral weakness is caused either by a nerve root lesion, especially C6 and C8, or by a lesion of the radial nerve.
• Bilateral weakness suggests either lead poisoning, or bronchus carcinoma, or a more general neurological disease.

Variation: resisted extension of the wrist with the fingers held actively flexed

Significance. This test can be used to differentiate between wrist extensors and finger extensors.

Active contraction of the finger flexors inhibits the finger extensors. Absence of pain indicates that, when a lesion is present, it lies in one of the finger extensors.

Positioning. The subject is standing and holds the extended arm forwards. He squeezes his bent fingers into the palm of his hand. The examiner stands level with the subject's arm and stabilizes the forearm with one hand. The other hand is placed at the dorsum of the subject's hand (Fig. 3.43).

Procedure. Resist the subject's attempt to extend the wrist.

Common mistakes:
- The entire arm is lifted up.
- The elbow is not held in extension.

Resisted radial deviation

Procedure. Resist the subject's attempt to move the hand radially (Fig. 3.44).

Common mistakes:
- The thumb is not left free, the result of which is that the thumb extensors and abductors become directly involved.
- The elbow is not kept extended.

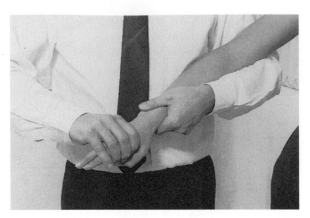

Fig. 3.44   Resisted radial deviation of the wrist.

Anatomical structures tested:

Muscle function:
- Extensor carpi radialis longus
- Abductor pollicis longus
- Extensor pollicis longus
- Flexor carpi radialis
- Flexor pollicis longus
- Brachioradialis

Neural function:

Muscle	Innervation	
	Peripheral	Nerve root
Extensor carpi radialis longus	Radial	C6–C7
Abductor pollicis longus	Radial	C7–C8
Extensor pollicis longus	Radial	C7–C8
Flexor carpi radialis	Median	C7–T1
Flexor pollicis longus	Median	C7–C8
Brachioradialis	Radial	C5–C8

Common pathological situations:
- Pain is most commonly present in tendinitis of either the extensor carpi radialis longus and / or brevis, or the flexor carpi radialis.
- The test may also be painful in de Quervain's tenovaginitis – a lesion of the abductor pollicis longus and extensor pollicis brevis in their common tendon sheath.

Resisted ulnar deviation

Procedure. Resist the subject's attempt to push the hand over to the ulnar side (Fig. 3.45).

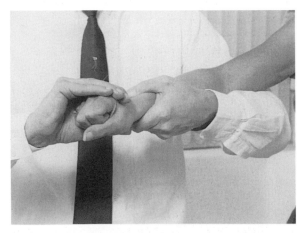

Fig. 3.43   Resisted extension of the wrist with fingers flexed.

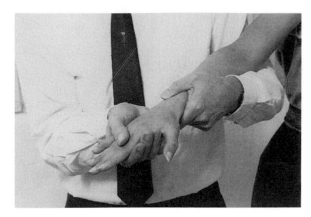

Fig. 3.45   Resisted ulnar deviation of the wrist.

Common mistakes. The elbow is not extended.

Anatomical structures tested:

Muscle function:
* *Important ulnar deviators*:
    – Extensor carpi ulnaris
    – Flexor carpi ulnaris
* *Less important ulnar deviators*:
    – Extensor digitorum communis
    – Extensor digiti minimi.

Neural function:

Muscle	Innervation	
	Peripheral	Nerve root
Extensor carpi ulnaris	Radial	C7–C8
Flexor carpi ulnaris	Ulnar	C7–C8
Extensor digitorum communis	Radial	C6–C8
Extensor digiti minimi	Radial	C6–C8

Common pathological situations:
* Pain is the result of tendinitis either of the extensor carpi ulnaris or of the flexor carpi ulnaris.
* Weakness indicates usually a C8 nerve root lesion.

Muscles controlling the thumb

Remarks

The positioning of the subject is the same for the four tests. So is the positioning of the examiner,

Box 3.1	Definitions
Adduction	The thumb moves from a palmar position dorsally to join the plane of the other metacarpals.
Abduction	The thumb moves in a palmar direction, away from the plane of the other metacarpals.
Extension	At carpometacarpal, metacarpophalangeal and interphalangeal joints there is a movement in the radial direction roughly in a plane parallel to the plane of the other metacarpals.
Flexion	At carpometacarpal, metacarpophalangeal and interphalangeal joints there is a movement in the ulnar direction roughly in a plane parallel to the plane of the other metacarpals.

except that for flexion and extension (see Box 3.1 for definitions) resistance is given at the distal phalanx and for abduction and adduction at the distal part (head) of the first metacarpal bone.

Positioning. The subject stands with the arm hanging, the elbow bent to a right angle, the forearm and hand in the neutral position, and the thumb pointing upwards. The examiner faces the subject. The contralateral hand carries the subject's wrist. The other hand is on the thumb.

Resisted flexion

Procedure. Resist the subject's attempt to flex the thumb (Fig. 3.46).

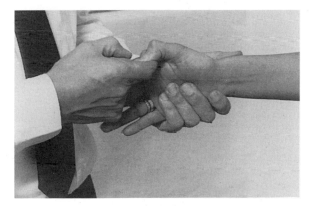

Fig. 3.46   Resisted flexion of the thumb.

Common mistakes. The thumb is allowed to hyperextend at the metacarpophalangeal joint.

Anatomical structures tested:

Muscle function:
- *Important thumb flexors*:
  - Flexor pollicis longus
  - Flexor pollicis brevis
- *Less important thumb flexor*:
  - Adductor pollicis.

Neural function:

Muscle	Innervation	
	Peripheral	Nerve root
Flexor pollicis longus	Median	C7–C8
Flexor pollicis brevis		
superficial head	Median	C8–T1
deep head	Ulnar	C8–T1
Adductor pollicis	Ulnar	C8–T1

Common pathological situations:
- Pain is present in a tenosynovitis of the flexor pollicis longus.
- Weakness is suggestive of a lesion of a branch of the median nerve – the anterior interosseous nerve – and, more rarely, of the ulnar nerve.

Resisted extension

Procedure. Resist the subject's attempt to extend the thumb (Fig. 3.47).

Common mistakes. Hyperextension of the first metacarpophalangeal joint takes place.

Anatomical structures tested:

Muscle function:
- Extensor pollicis longus
- Extensor pollicis brevis
- Abductor pollicis longus.

Neural function:

Muscle	Innervation	
	Peripheral	Nerve root
Extensor pollicis longus	Radial	C7–C8
Extensor pollicis brevis	Radial	C7–T1
Abductor pollicis longus	Radial	C7–C8

Common pathological situations:
- Pain occurs in tendinous lesions of the abductor pollicis longus and extensor pollicis brevis (de Quervain's disease) and extensor pollicis longus (crepitating tenosynovitis).
- Weakness is possibly the result of a rupture of the extensor pollicis longus. It may also indicate a neurological condition, either of the radial nerve or of the C8 nerve root.

Resisted abduction

Procedure. Resist the subject's attempt to abduct the thumb (Fig. 3.48).

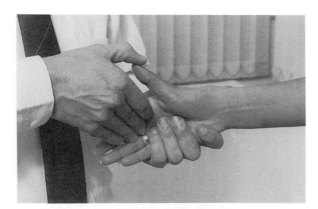

Fig. 3.47 Resisted extension of the thumb.

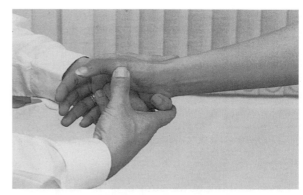

Fig. 3.48 Resisted abduction of the thumb.

Common mistakes. Resistance is given on the distal phalanx.

Anatomical structures tested:

Muscle function:
• Abductor pollicis longus
• Abductor pollicis brevis
• Extensor pollicis brevis
• (Flexor pollicis brevis).

Neural function:

Muscle	Innervation	
	Peripheral	Nerve root
Abductor pollicis longus	Radial	C7–C8
Abductor pollicis brevis	Median	C8–T1
Extensor pollicis brevis	Radial	C7–T1
(Flexor pollicis brevis, deep head	Ulnar	C8–T1)

Common pathological situations:
• Pain is the result of a tendinous lesion of the abductor pollicis longus and extensor pollicis brevis, e.g. de Quervain's disease, or crepitating tenosynovitis.
• Weakness occurs in nerve lesions, e.g. posterior interosseous nerve or median nerve.

Resisted adduction

Procedure. Resist the subject's attempt to adduct the thumb (Fig. 3.49).

Common mistakes. Resistance is given at the distal phalanx.

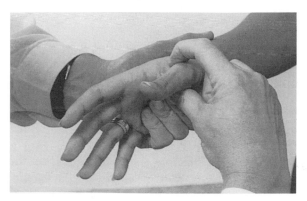

Fig. 3.49 Resisted adduction of the thumb.

Anatomical structures tested:

Muscle function:
• *Important thumb adductor:*
  – Adductor pollicis
• *Less important thumb adductors:*
  – Flexor pollicis brevis, superficial head
  – Opponens pollicis.

Neural function:

Muscle	Innervation	
	Peripheral	Nerve root
Adductor pollicis	Ulnar	C8–T1
Flexor pollicis brevis superficial head	Median	C8–T1
Opponens pollicis	Median	C6–C7

Common pathological situations:
• Pain occurs in a lesion of the adductor pollicis, usually in the oblique portion.
• Weakness occurs in lesions of either the ulnar nerve or the C8 nerve root.

Muscles controlling the fingers

Resisted extension of each finger separately

Positioning and procedure. The subject presents his hand palm downwards. The examiner stabilizes the wrist with one hand. With the other, he applies resistance to the distal phalanx of each finger respectively (Fig. 3.50).

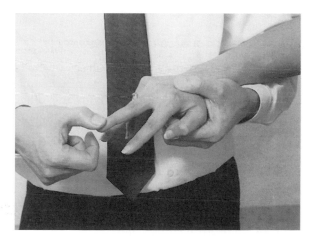

Fig. 3.50 Resisted extension of one finger.

Common mistakes. None.

Anatomical structures tested:

Muscle function:
- Extension of the index finger:
  - Extensor indicis proprius
  - Tendon to the index finger of the extensor digitorum communis muscle
- Extension of the middle finger:
  - Tendon to the middle finger of the extensor digitorum communis muscle
- Extension of the ring finger:
  - Tendon to the ring finger of the extensor digitorum communis muscle
- Extension of the little finger:
  - Extensor digiti minimi
  - Tendon to the little finger of the extensor digitorum communis muscle.

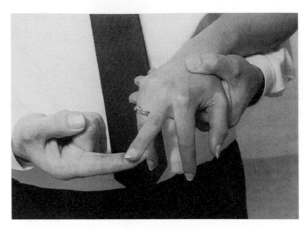

Fig. 3.51   Resisted flexion of one finger.

Neural function:

Muscle	Innervation	
	Peripheral	Nerve root
Extensor indicis proprius	Radial	C6–C8
Extensor digitorum communis	Radial	C6–C8
Extensor digiti minimi	Radial	C6–C8

Neural function:

Muscle	Innervation	
	Peripheral	Nerve root
Flexor digitorum superficialis	Median	C7–T1
Flexor digitorum profundus	Median	C7–T1

Common pathological situations:
- Pain occurs in tendinitis of the extensor indicis proprius or of one of the tendons of the extensor digitorum communis.
- Weakness may occur in a lesion of the radial nerve.

Resisted flexion of each finger separately

Positioning and procedure. The subject presents his hand palm downwards. The examiner stabilizes the wrist with one hand. With the other hand he applies resistance to the distal phalanx of each finger respectively (Fig. 3.51).

Common mistakes. None.

Anatomical structures tested:

Muscle function:
- Flexor digitorum superficialis
- Flexor digitorum profundus.

Common pathological situations:
- When resisted movement of one specific finger is painful, the lesion, if present, must lie in the tendon going to that finger.
- Pain is usually the result of a lesion of one of the tendons of the flexor digitorum profundus, either at the wrist or more distally.

Intrinsic muscles of the hand

Remark

When the intrinsic muscles of the hand are affected, it is usually a lesion in the dorsal interossei. These muscles mainly abduct the fingers away from the middle finger (Fig. 3.52, left).

There are four dorsal interossei and three palmar ones. The latter adduct the fingers towards the middle finger (Fig. 3.52, right).

These muscles can be tested by spreading the fingers against resistance followed by squeezing the examiner's finger. The combination of positive answers indicates which muscle is affected.

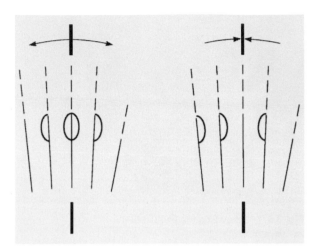

Fig. 3.52 (Left) Abduction, four dorsal interossei; (right) adduction, three palmar interossei.

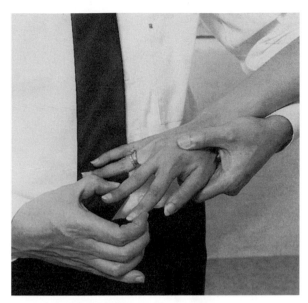

Fig. 3.53 Resisted separation of the fingers: II–III.

The positioning is the same for all six tests. When spreading the examiner applics resistance at the distal phalanges. During squeezing the examiner places his finger between the proximal interphalangeal joints.

There are no common mistakes.

Spreading: II–III

Procedure. Resist the subject's attempt to spread the index and middle fingers (Fig. 3.53).

Anatomical structures tested:

Muscle function:
- Interosseus dorsalis I
- Interosseus dorsalis III.

Spreading: III–IV

Procedure. Resist the subject's attempt to spread the middle and ring fingers (Fig. 3.54).

Anatomical structures tested:

Muscle function:
- Interosseus dorsalis II
- Interosseus dorsalis IV.

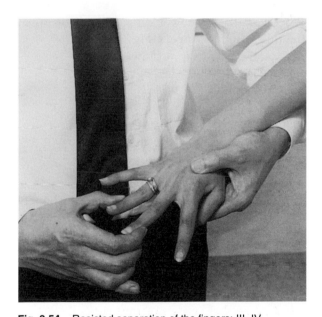

Fig. 3.54 Resisted separation of the fingers: III–IV.

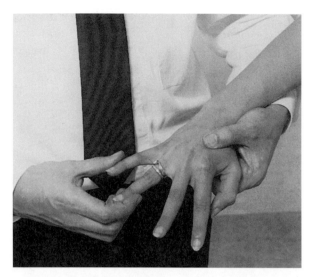

Fig. 3.55 Resisted separation of the fingers: IV–V.

Spreading: IV–V

Procedure. Resist the subject's attempt to spread the ring and little fingers (Fig. 3.55).

Anatomical structures tested:

Muscle function:
- Interosseus palmaris IV
- Abductor digiti minimi.

Squeezing: II–III

Procedure. Resist the subject's attempt to squeeze your finger between index and middle fingers (Fig. 3.56).

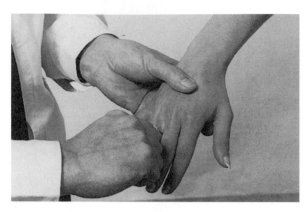

Fig. 3.57 Squeezing the fingers: III–IV.

Anatomical structures tested:

Muscle function:
- Interosseus palmaris II
- Interosseus dorsalis II.

Squeezing: III–IV

Procedure. Resist the subject's attempt to squeeze your finger between middle and ring fingers (Fig. 3.57).

Anatomical structures tested:

Muscle function:
- Interosseus dorsalis III
- Interosseus palmaris IV.

Squeezing: IV–V

Procedure. Resist the subject's attempt to squeeze your finger between ring and little fingers (Fig. 3.58).

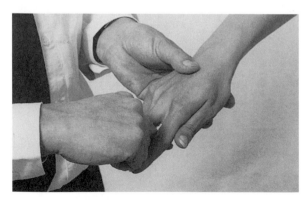

Fig. 3.56 Squeezing the fingers: II–III.

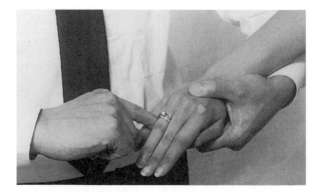

Fig. 3.58 Squeezing the fingers: IV–V.

Anatomical structures tested:

Muscle function:
- Interosseus dorsalis IV
- Interosseus palmaris V.

Neural function:

Muscle	Innervation	
	Peripheral	Nerve root
Dorsal interossei	Ulnar	C8–T1
Palmar interossei	Ulnar	C8–T1
Abductor digiti minimi	Ulnar	C8–T1

Common pathological situations:
- Pain is usually the result of a lesion in one of the dorsal interossei. The combination of positive tests shows which one is affected.
- Weakness may be one of the first signs of an amyotrophic lateral sclerosis or of involvement of the T1 nerve root. It may also indicate a lesion of the ulnar nerve.

SPECIFIC TESTS
Phalen's test = forced flexion of the wrist (Fig. 3.59)

Significance. This is a compression test for the median nerve in the carpal tunnel. Release of the pressure causes paraesthesia in the territory of the median nerve – 3½ fingers medially and palmar.

Positioning. The subject presents the hand. The examiner grasps the distal forearm with the contralateral hand. With the other hand he takes hold of the subject's hand.

Procedure. Bring the subject's wrist passively into full flexion and keep it in that position for about a minute. Then suddenly release the compression.

Tinel's test = percussion of the carpal tunnel (Fig. 3.60)

Significance. This is a percussion test for the median nerve in the carpal tunnel or for the ulnar nerve in Guyon's tunnel. It should elicit paraesthesia in the territory either of the median nerve – 3½ fingers medially and palmar, or of the ulnar nerve – 1½ ulnar fingers.

Positioning. The subject presents the hand palm upwards. The examiner grasps the wrist with one hand. The other hand uses the percussion hammer.

Procedure. Give a slight percussion on the carpal tunnel.
Give a slight percussion on Guyon's tunnel.

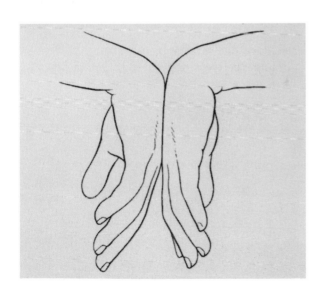

Fig. 3.59 Phalen's test.

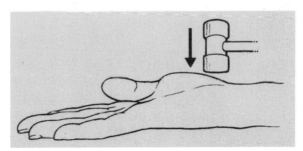

Fig. 3.60 Tinel's test.

Grind test for the trapezium–first metacarpal joint (Fig. 3.61)

Significance. This test is meant to detect crepitus as a symptom indicating arthrosis.

Positioning. The subject stands with the arm hanging and the elbow 90° flexed. The examiner stands level with the subject's hand. The contralateral hand grasps and stabilizes the wrist. The other hand takes hold of the distal part of the first metacarpal bone.

Procedure. Exert axial pressure and circumduct the first metacarpal bone.

Finkelstein's test (Fig. 3.62)

Significance. This test is meant to confirm the presence of de Quervain's disease. It should be more painful than the ulnar deviation test as described on page 51.

Positioning. The subject stands with the arm hanging, the elbow flexed to a right angle and the forearm pronated. The examiner stands next to the subject. The contralateral hand carries the forearm, which is kept between his arm and trunk. The other hand grasps the subject's hand distally on the metacarpals, first metacarpal included.

Procedure. Pull the subject's wrist to the ulnar side until the end of range is reached.

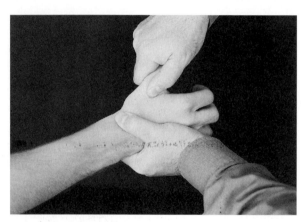

Fig. 3.61 Grind test.

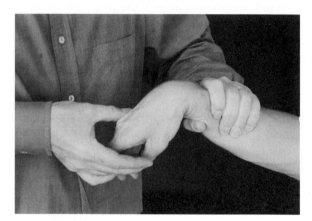

Fig. 3.62 Finkelstein's test.

4

Hip

SURFACE AND PALPATORY ANATOMY

ANTERIOR

Bony landmarks (Fig. 4.1)

The inguinal fold can easily be identified. It covers the inguinal ligament (A) that can be palpated as a strong fibrous band.

The anterior superior iliac spine (B) is located at the craniolateral end of the fold. This bony prominence forms the point of origin of both the sartorius muscle and the tensor fasciae latae

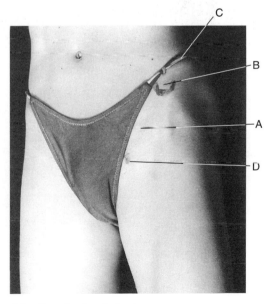

Fig. 4.1   Bony landmarks in vivo.

muscles. The spine continues laterally and dorsally in the iliac crest (C).

At the medial end of the inguinal fold another bony prominence can be palpated, the pubic tubercle (D). Normally it lies level with the superior aspect of the greater trochanter. It provides attachment for the medial end of the inguinal ligament and for the tendon of the rectus abdominis. The tendon of the adductor longus originates just below this tubercle.

Palpation of soft tissue

Palpation of the superficial flexors: the lateral femoral triangle (Fig. 4.2)

Place the palpating finger a few centimetres distal to the anterior superior iliac spine and ask the patient to lift and abduct the extended leg. Two structures can be felt and/or seen, one at each side of the finger, forming an inverted V (the lateral femoral triangle). The sartorius (A) is the medial and the tensor fasciae latae the lateral muscle (B) (Fig. 4.3). Notice also the belly of the rectus femoris (C) a few centimetres distal to the inverted V (Fig. 4.4).

The origin of the latter is felt deeply in the lateral femoral triangle, about 5 cm distal to the anterior superior iliac spine. Ask the patient to extend the knee, bend the hip to 60° and add some resistance. This movement makes the belly of the muscle better visible. Palpate a bony prominence – the inferior iliac spine – from which the muscle originates.

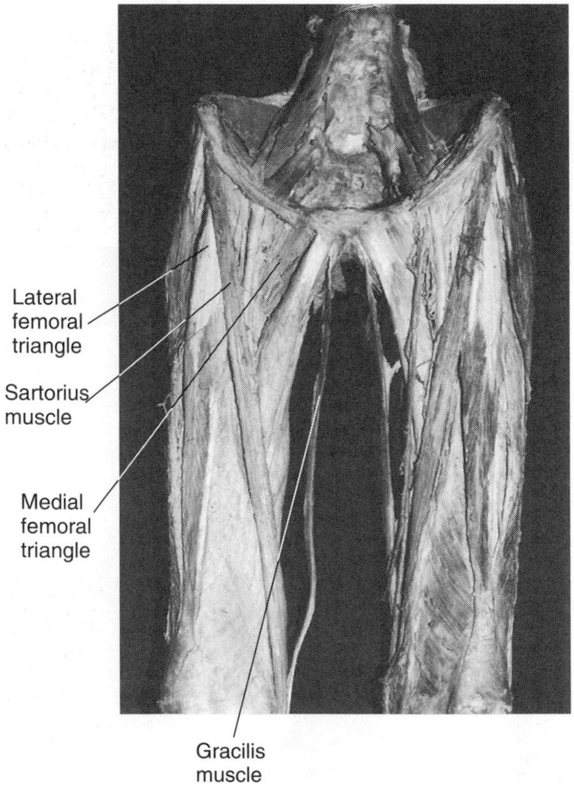

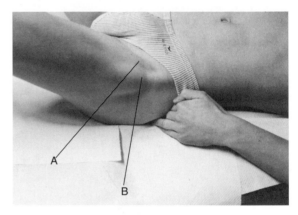

Fig. 4.3 Lateral femoral triangle.

Lateral femoral triangle

Sartorius muscle

Medial femoral triangle

Gracilis muscle

Fig. 4.2 Bony landmarks.

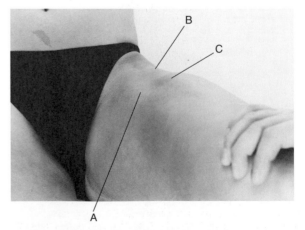

Fig. 4.4 Rectus femoris in the lateral femoral triangle.

Medial femoral triangle (trigonum of Scarpa)
(Fig. 4.5)

The medial femoral triangle is defined superiorly by the inguinal ligament, medially by the adductor longus and laterally by the sartorius. The floor of the triangle is formed by portions of the iliopsoas on the lateral side and the pectineus on the medial side.

Definition in vivo

To define the belly of the sartorius. Stand level with the knee of the subject at the ipsilateral side and face the hip. The hip is slightly bent and slightly abducted. Keep the knee 90° flexed with its lateral side resting against your hip.

Ask the patient to perform a flexion and lateral rotation at the hip. The former is resisted with the contralateral hand, the latter with the ipsilateral one. The muscle becomes even more visible if the subject is asked to add some flexion movement in the knee (Fig. 4.6).

To define the adductor longus. The starting position is the same. Stand level with the slightly flexed knee. The hip is slightly flexed and abducted, the foot rests on the couch.

Place the ipsilateral hand at the inner side of the knee and resist the adduction movement. The adductor longus is revealed as the most prominent anterior and medial structure (Fig. 4.7).

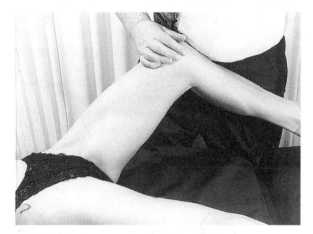

Fig. 4.6   Palpation of sartorius (muscle).

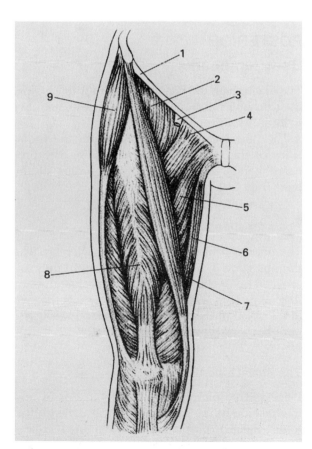

Fig. 4.5   Anterior view of the hip muscle: 1, inguinal ligament; 2, iliopsoas; 3, femoral artery; 4, pectineus; 5, adductor longus; 6, gracilis; 7, sartorius; 8, rectus femoris; 9, tensor fasciae latae.

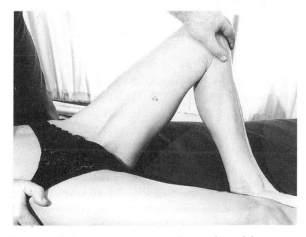

Fig. 4.7   Palpation of the adductor longus (muscle).

Palpation of the iliopsoas tendon and neurovascular structures in the groin

The most important landmark is the femoral artery whose pulse is easily found under the inguinal ligament. The artery courses downwards and slightly medially towards the tip of the triangle.

The femoral nerve can sometimes be felt as a small and round strand rolling under the palpating finger about one finger-width lateral to the artery and just distal to the inguinal ligament.

The femoral vein is medial to the artery and in normal circumstances not palpable.

The tendon of the iliopsoas can be detected between the femoral artery and the sartorius muscle, just below the inguinal ligament. To facilitate the palpation one can bring the hip into slight flexion and slight lateral rotation. The localization can be confirmed when the patient is asked to flex the hip against resistance.

The muscular structure that can be palpated deeply in the medial corner of the medial femoral triangle is the pectineus muscle. Just medial to it the strong adductor longus is again recognized.

Palpation of the long adductors

Muscle bellies of adductor longus, gracilis and adductor magnus can be palpated at the medial side of the thigh. They take origin from the pubic tubercle (adductor longus) and the ischiopubic ramus (gracilis and adductor magnus).

The structure that becomes visible during passive abduction of the hip is the adductor longus (Fig. 4.8, A). Its origin at the pubic tubercle can be palpated as a strong cord (Fig. 4.7).

Posterior to the adductor longus and slightly more lateral the gracilis (B) can be palpated. As this is a bi-articular structure it becomes more stretched when the knee is extended during a passive hip abduction. The broad and flat tendon on the ischiopubic ramus is therefore felt to press against the palpating finger when the knee of the abducted leg is gradually brought into extension.

The origin of the adductor magnus is posterior to the gracilis and anterior to the origin of the hamstrings on the ischial tuberosity. The muscle

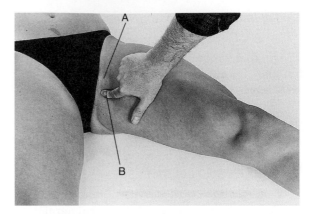

Fig. 4.8 Palpation of the gracilis.

is only palpable over a small extent and therefore difficult to examine.

POSTERIOR

Bony landmarks

The iliac crests, the posterior superior iliac spine, the trochanter and the ischial tuberosity are easy to locate in a prone lying subject.

The iliac crests are palpated with the radial sides of the index fingers by holding the pronated hands against the lower borders of the loins (Fig. 4.9).

Posterior superior iliac spine

The pronated hands rest on the iliac crests. The thumbs glide in a caudal direction until they are arrested by the bony and thick posterior superior iliac spine (Fig. 4.9). In most individuals the lack of fat tissue at this level can be seen as a dimple just above and medial to the buttock.

The ischial tuberosity

Place the palpating thumbs at the dorsal and medial side of the thighs, well below the gluteal folds (Fig. 4.10), and move them in a cranial direction. The first bone that is encountered is the ischial tuberosity. It provides attachment for the hamstring tendons posteriorly and the quadratus femoris and adductor magnus medially.

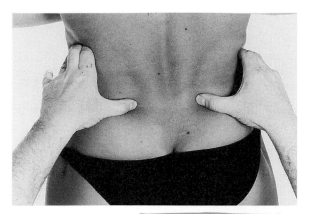

Fig. 4.9 Palpation of the posterior superior iliac spines.

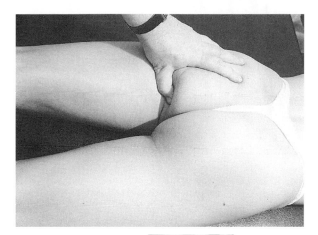

Fig. 4.10 Palpation of the ischial tuberosity.

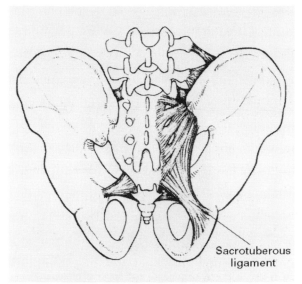

Fig. 4.11 The sacrotuberous ligament.

With the hip extended, the tuberosity is covered by the gluteus maximus and adipose tissue. If the hip is flexed, the gluteus maximus moves upwards and the ischial tuberosity becomes better palpable. At the medial aspect of the tuberosity a strong fibrous band can be felt, joining the sacrum in a craniomedial direction. This is the sacrotuberous ligament (Fig. 4.11).

Trochanter (Fig. 4.12)

Palpation of this important landmark is relatively easy at its posterior edge, where the bone is not covered by muscles. The upper aspect of both trochanters should be on the same horizontal

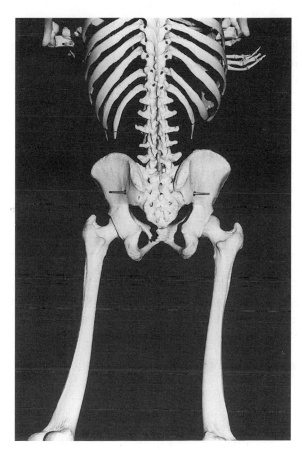

Fig. 4.12 Localization of the trochanters.

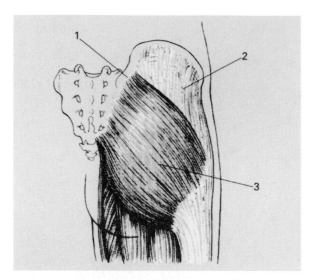

Fig. 4.13 1, Posterior superior iliac spine; 2, gluteus medius; 3, gluteus maximus.

level as the pubic tubercles, the coccyx and the head of the femur.

Palpation of soft tissue

Gluteus maximus (Fig. 4.13)

The muscle belly of the gluteus maximus and fat deposits are responsible for the typical shape of the buttocks. The muscle is palpable over its entire width. Extension of the thigh brings it into a contracted position. The upper border of the muscle coincides with the line connecting the upper border of the trochanter with the upper border of the posterior superior iliac spine. The lower border of the muscle is not the lower border of the gluteal fold as the latter consists merely of fat tissue.

Gluteus medius (Fig. 4.14)

Only a small part of the muscle can be palpated between the iliac crest, the upper border of the trochanter, the upper border of the gluteus maximus and the posterior border of the tensor fascia lata.

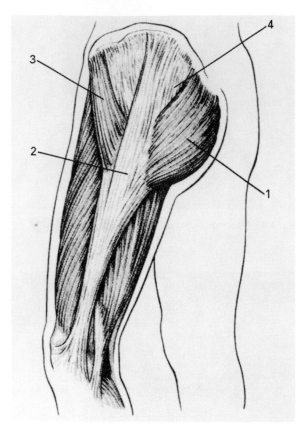

Fig. 4.14 Lateral view of the hip muscles: 1, gluteus maximus; 2, iliotibial tract; 3, tensor fasciae latae; 4, gluteus medius.

Hamstrings (Figs 4.15 and 4.16)

Biceps, semitendinosus and semimembranosus originate from a common tendon at the inferior aspect of the ischial tuberosity. If the hip is slightly flexed, the gluteus maximus moves upwards, exposing the ischial tuberosity so the tendon can be palpated more easily. A resisted flexion of the knee makes it visible.

Sciatic nerve (Fig. 4.17)

The sciatic nerve passes to the leg between the greater trochanter and the ischial tuberosity. In a slightly flexed position of the hip, this nerve is palpable underneath the adipose tissue.

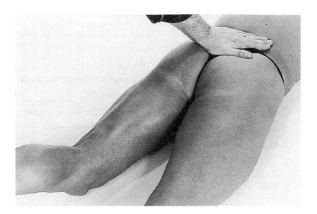

Fig. 4.15   Palpation of the hamstrings.

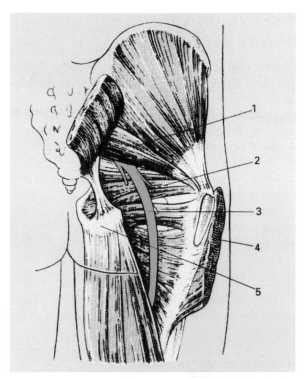

Fig. 4.17   The sciatic nerve: 1, piriformis; 2, gemellus superior; 3, sciatic nerve; 4, gluteus maximus (resected); 5, ischial tuberosity.

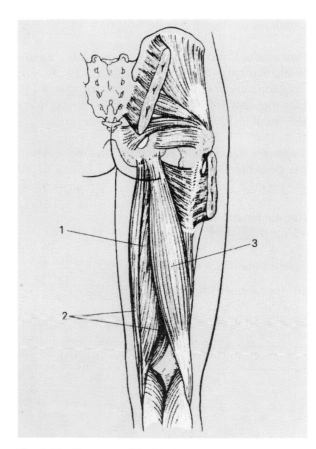

Fig. 4.16   Extensors of the hip (hamstrings): 1, semitendinosus; 2, semimembranosus; 3, biceps femoris.

FUNCTIONAL EXAMINATION OF THE HIP

Introduction/general remarks

Examination of the hip cannot be disconnected from that of the lumbar spine and the sacroiliac joints: pain in the buttock or thigh has very often a lumbar or sacroiliac origin. Furthermore, it is also very difficult to examine the hip without applying stress on sacroiliac joints and lumbar joints.

Therefore, a preliminary examination of lumbar spine and sacroiliac joint may be appropriate to exclude any lesion in these regions.

Most of the hip tests are executed by using the leg as a lever.

PASSIVE TESTS

Passive flexion

Positioning. The subject lies relaxed in the supine position. The examiner stands level with the hip.

Procedure. Both hands lift the knee upwards towards the subject's chest until the movement stops. Meanwhile a slight axial pressure is applied on the femur (Fig. 4.18).

Common mistakes:
- Moving the thigh too much laterally towards the shoulder.
- Carrying the movement too far, beyond the range where the tilt of the pelvis starts. This is precluded by sufficient axial pressure.

Alternative technique: one hand can be placed under the pelvis in order to detect the start of the pelvic tilt.

Normal functional anatomy:
- *Range*: 110–130°
- *End-feel*: ligamentous
- *Limiting structures*:
  - posterior part of the joint capsule
  - muscles of the buttock
  - contact between labrum and neck.

Common pathological situations:
- Too hard an end-feel on passive flexion is one of the first signs of an osteoarthrosis.
- In advanced arthrosis this movement is markedly limited. Typically the femur moves laterally when the flexion is forced.
- In children this abduction movement during flexion is often the first manifestation of Perthes' disease.

Passive external rotation

Positioning. The subject lies in the supine position with the hip and knee bent to 90°. The examiner stands level with the subject's hip. One hand supports the lower leg just above the ankle, the other hand is put at the knee and stabilizes the femur in a vertical position.

Procedure. Rotate the lower leg inwards, meanwhile assuring the vertical position of the femur, until the movement comes to a soft stop (Fig. 4.19). Observe the anterior iliac spine of the opposite side to detect the start of a lateral pelvic tilt.

Common mistakes. The leg is pushed beyond the possible range, which causes a lateral tilt of the pelvis.

Normal functional anatomy:
- *Range*: 60–90°

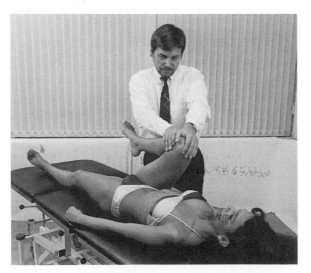

Fig. 4.18 Passive flexion.

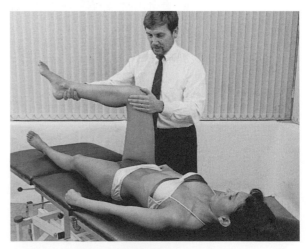

Fig. 4.19 Passive external rotation.

- *End-feel*: ligamentous
- *Limiting structures*:
  - superior part of the iliofemoral ligament
  - pubofemoral ligament
  - tensor fasciae latae and gluteus minimus

Common pathological situations:
- This movement can be extremely painful and/or limited in psoas bursitis, trochanteric bursitis and in the presence of internal derangement in the hip.
- Children with a slipped epiphysis may present with an increased range of external rotation.
- In arthrosis the external rotation is usually the last movement to become disturbed.

Passive medial rotation

Positioning. The subject lies in the supine position with the hip and knee bent to 90°. The examiner stands level with the subject's hip. One hand supports the lower leg just above the ankle, the other hand stabilizes the femur at the knee.

Procedure. Rotate the lower leg outwards, meanwhile assuring the vertical position of the femur, until the movement comes to a soft stop (Fig. 4.20).

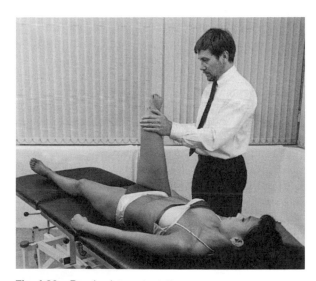

Fig. 4.20 Passive internal rotation.

Observe the anterior iliac spine of the opposite side to detect the start of a lateral pelvic tilt.

Common mistakes. The movement is continued beyond the possible range, which causes a lateral tilt of the pelvis.

Normal functional anatomy:
- *Range*: 45–60°
- *End-feel*: ligamentous
- *Limiting structures*:
  - the ischiofemoral ligament
  - buttock muscles: gluteus maximus, gluteus medius, piriformis, gemelli, obturator externus and internus, quadratus femoris.

Common pathological situations:
- In arthritis, the medial rotation is the most painful movement.
- In arthrosis it is usually the first movement to become limited.

Passive abduction

Positioning. The subject lies in the supine position, near the border of the couch, with the lower leg pendent. The examiner stands level with the subject's hip. One hand grasps the distal thigh from the medial side. The other hand is placed on the opposite anterior superior iliac spine in order to stabilize the pelvis.

Procedure. The knee is abducted with the pendent lower leg until the movement stops (Fig. 4.21).

Common mistakes:
- Carrying on abduction beyond the start of the lateral pelvic tilt.
- Owing to tension in the bi-articular gracilis, abduction with extended knee has very often a shorter range of motion.

Normal functional anatomy:
- *Range*: 45–60°
- *End-feel*: hard ligamentous
- *Limiting structures*:
  - pubofemoral and ischiofemoral ligaments
  - adductor muscles.

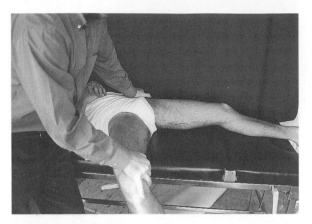

Fig. 4.21 Passive abduction.

Common pathological situations:
- This test may provoke groin pain in an adductor tendinitis and trochanteric or gluteal pain in bursitis.
- Serious painful limitation occurs in arthritis and painless limitation in arthrosis.

Passive adduction

Positioning. The subject lies in a relaxed supine position. The examiner stands at the foot-end of the couch. One hand carries the heel, the other hand lifts the extended contralateral leg to about 45° of flexion.

Procedure. Move the leg into adduction under the extended contralateral leg until the pelvis starts tilting laterally (Fig. 4.22).

Common mistakes:
- Carrying on adduction beyond the start of lateral pelvic tilt.
- Adduction and medial rotation is unintentionally added in the contralateral hip.

Normal functional anatomy:
- *Range*: 20–45°
- *End-feel*: soft ligamentous
- *Limiting structures*:
  - superior part of the iliofemoral ligament
  - iliotibial band, tensor fasciae latae superior part of gluteus maximus and medius, gemelli, piriformis and obturator internus.

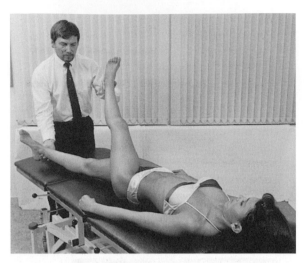

Fig. 4.22 Passive adduction.

Common pathological situations. When the movement is painful at the outer side of the hip, a lesion of the iliotibial tract or a gluteal bursitis may be considered.

Passive extension

Positioning. The subject lies prone with the hip extended. The examiner stands level with the hip. One hand is placed on the thigh, just below the gluteal fold. The other hand grasps the thigh just proximal to the patella.

Procedure. Lift the knee off the couch until the movement comes to a stop. Meanwhile press the pelvis firmly to the couch (Fig. 4.23).

Common mistakes:
- Lack of stabilization allows the pelvis to move upwards, causing a false interpretation of the range of hip extension and putting stress on the lower lumbar spine and the sacroiliac joint.
- If the stabilizing hand is placed too high up on the sacrum, stress will be induced at the ipsilateral sacroiliac joint.

Normal functional anatomy:
- *Range*: 10–30°
- *End-feel*: hard ligamentous

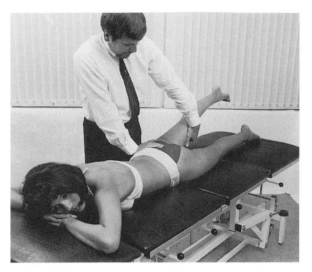

Fig. 4.23   Passive extension.

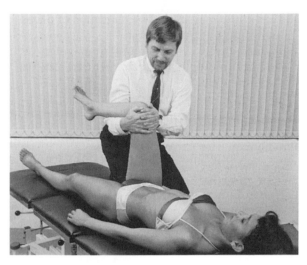

Fig. 4.24   Resisted flexion.

- *Limiting structures*:
  – anterior part of the capsule with the iliofemoral, pubofemoral and ischiofemoral ligaments
  – iliopsoas muscle.

Common pathological situations:
- Extension is one of the first movements to become restricted in 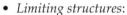arthritis and arthrosis.
- Some children have an isolated limitation of extension.

ISOMETRIC CONTRACTIONS
Resisted flexion

Positioning. The subject lies in the supine position with the hip flexed to a right angle. The examiner stands level with the thigh and places one knee against the ischial tuberosity. Both hands are clasped at the anterior and distal end of the thigh.

Procedure. Resist the subject's attempt to flex the hip (Fig. 4.24).

Common mistakes. A sudden start or sudden stop may induce unintentional movement.

Anatomical structures tested:

Muscle function:
- *Important flexors*:
  – Iliopsoas
  – Rectus femoris
  – Sartorius
  – Tensor fasciae latae
- *Accessory flexors*:
  – Pectineus
  – Adductor longus, brevis and magnus.

Neural function:

Muscle	Innervation	
	Peripheral	Nerve root
Iliopsoas	Femoral nerve + lumbar plexus	L2, L3
Sartorius	Femoral nerve	L2, L3
Rectus femoris	Femoral nerve	L3
Tensor fasciae latae	Superior gluteal nerve	L5
Pectineus	Femoral + obturator nerve	L2, L3
Adductor longus	Obturator nerve	L2, L3
Adductor brevis	Obturator nerve	L2, L3
Adductor magnus	Obturator + sciatic nerve	L3, L4

Common pathological situations:
- A painless weakness is always a warning sign for serious disorders: second root palsy, nervus femoralis palsy or abdominal neoplasma. It may, however, also be present in psychoneurosis.

- Pain alone may indicate a tendinitis of psoas, sartorius or rectus femoris.
- Pain and weakness are found in avulsion fractures of the lesser trochanter and anterior superior spine.

Resisted abduction

Positioning. The subject lies supine and relaxed with both hips slightly abducted. The examiner stands at the foot-end of the couch and places both hands on the lateral aspect of the lower legs, just proximal to the ankles.

Procedure. Resist the abduction movement (Fig. 4.25).

Common mistakes. None.

Anatomical structures tested:

Muscle function:
- *Important abductors*:
  - Gluteus medius
  - Gluteus minimus
  - Tensor fasciae latae
  - Gluteus maximus
- *Accessory abductors*:
  - Piriformis
  - Sartorius.

Neural function:

Muscle	Innervation	
	Peripheral	Nerve root
Gluteus medius	Superior gluteal nerve	L5
Gluteus minimus	Superior gluteal nerve	L5
Tensor fasciae latae	Superior gluteal nerve	L5
Gluteus maximus (upper part)	Inferior gluteal nerve	S1
Piriformis	Lumbosacral plexus	S1, S2
Sartorius	Femoral nerve	L2, L3

Common pathological situations:
- Pain may be the result of compression of an inflamed gluteal bursa.
- Alternatively it may originate from stress placed upon strained or inflamed sacroiliac ligaments.
- In congenital dislocation of the hip the movement shows some weakness.

Resisted adduction

Positioning. The subject lies supine and relaxed with both hips slightly abducted. The examiner stands at the foot-end of the couch and places the clenched fist between both knees (Fig. 4.26).

Procedure. Ask the subject to squeeze the fist.

Common mistakes. None.

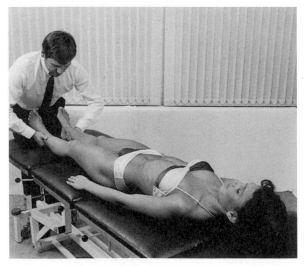

Fig. 4.25 Resisted abduction.

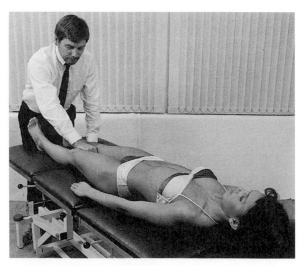

Fig. 4.26 Resisted adduction.

Anatomical structures tested:

Muscle function:
- *Important adductors*:
  - Adductor longus
  - Adductor brevis
  - Adductor magnus
  - Pectineus
- *Accessory adductors*:
  - Gracilis
  - Gluteus maximus (lower part)
  - Obturator externus
  - Quadratus femoris
  - Biceps femoris.

Neural function:

Muscle	Innervation	
	Peripheral	Nerve root
Adductor longus	Obturator nerve	L2, L3
Adductor brevis	Obturator nerve	L2, L3
Adductor magnus	Obturator + sciatic nerve	L3, L4
Pectineus	Femoral + obturator nerve	L2, L3
Gracilis	Obturator nerve	L2, L3, L4
Gluteus maximus (lower part)	Inferior gluteal nerve	S1
Obturator externus	Obturator nerve	L3, L4
Quadratus femoris	Inferior gluteal nerve	L4, L5, S1
Biceps femoris	Sciatic nerve	S1, S2

Common pathological situations:
- Groin pain is usually the result of an adductor tendinitis or a stress fracture of the inferior pubic ramus.
- Buttock pain is often the consequence of transmitted stress to inflamed sacroiliac joints.

Resisted extension

Positioning. The subject lies in a relaxed supine position with the hips slightly abducted. The examiner stands at the foot-end of the couch. His clasped hands carry the heel and lift up the leg (Fig. 4.27).

Procedure. Ask the subject to push the extended leg towards the couch and resist the movement.

Common mistakes. None.

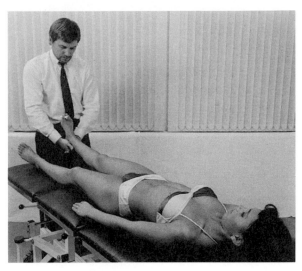

Fig. 4.27 Resisted extension.

Anatomical structures tested:

Muscle function:
- Gluteus maximus
- Semimembranosus
- Semitendinosus
- Biceps femoris
- Adductor magnus

Neural function:

Muscle	Innervation	
	Peripheral	Spinal
Gluteus maximus	Inferior gluteal nerve	S1
Semimembranosus	Sciatic nerve	S1, S2
Semitendinosus	Sciatic nerve	S1, S2
Biceps femoris	Sciatic nerve	S1, S2
Adductor magnus	Obturator + sciatic nerve	L3, L4

Common pathological situations. Pain may result from a hamstring lesion or a sacroiliac strain.

Resisted medial rotation

Positioning. The subject lies in the prone position with the hips slightly abducted and the knees flexed to 90°. The examiner sits at the foot-end of the couch, just distal to the knees, and places both hands against the outer malleoli.

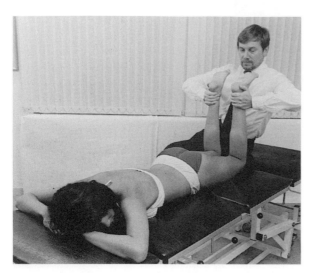

Fig. 4.28 Bilateral resisted medial rotation.

Procedure. Ask the subject to push the legs in an outward direction, and resist the movement (Fig. 4.28).

Common mistakes:
- Abduction of the thighs. Make sure that the knees do not separate during the procedure.
- Lordosis of the back. This could provoke pain from either the lumbosacral junction or the sacroiliac joints.

Anatomical structures tested:

Muscle function:
- Tensor fasciae latae
- Gluteus medius
- Gluteus minimus
- Adductor magnus.

Neural function:

Muscle	Innervation	
	Peripheral	Spinal
Tensor fasciae latae	Superior gluteal nerve	L5
Gluteus medius	Superior gluteal nerve	L5
Gluteus minimus	Superior gluteal nerve	L5
Adductor magnus	Obturator + sciatic nerve	L3, L4

Common pathological situations. Pain usually

results from transmitted stress to an inflamed bursa.

Resisted lateral rotation

Positioning. The subject lies prone with the hips slightly abducted and the knees flexed to 90°. The examiner sits at the foot-end of the couch, just distal to the knees. With crossed arms, he places both hands against the internal malleoli.

Procedure. Ask the subject to push the feet towards each other, and resist the movement (Fig. 4.29).

Common mistakes. Lordosis of the back may provoke pain from either the lumbosacral junction or the sacroiliac joints.

Anatomical structures tested:

Muscle function:
- *Important lateral rotators*:
  - Piriformis
  - Quadratus femoris
  - Obturator internus and externus
  - Gemelli
  - Gluteus medius and maximus
  - Sartorius
  - Iliopsoas

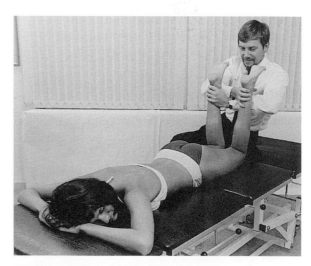

Fig. 4.29 Bilateral resisted lateral rotation.

- *Accessory lateral rotators*:
  - Adductor longus and brevis
  - Pectineus.

Neural function:

Muscle	Innervation	
	Peripheral	Spinal
Quadratus femoris	Sacral plexus	L4, L5, S1
Piriformis	Lumbosacral plexus	S1, S2
Obturator internus	Sacral plexus	L5, S1, S2
Obturator externus	Obturator nerve	L3, L4
Gemellus superior	Superior gluteal nerve	L5, S1
Gemellus inferior	Inferior gluteal nerve	L5, S1
Gluteus medius	Superior gluteal nerve	L4, L5, S1
Gluteus maximus	Inferior gluteal nerve	L5, S1, S2
Sartorius	Femoral nerve	L2, L3
Iliopsoas	Femoral nerve	L2, L3
Adductor brevis	Obturator nerve	L3, L4
Adductor longus	Obturator nerve	L3, L4
Pectineus	Femoral nerve	L2, L3

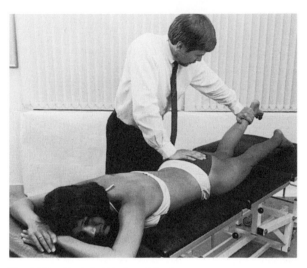

Fig. 4.30   Resisted flexion of the knee.

Common pathological situations:
- Gluteal pain is usually the result of a compression of an inflamed bursa.
- Groin pain may be provoked in lesions of the sartorius muscle.

Resisted flexion of the knee

Positioning. The subject lies prone with the knee in 30° of flexion. The examiner stands level with the thigh and leans over the subject. One hand is on the ilium, the other presses against the distal end of the lower leg.

Procedure. Ask the subject to flex the knee, and resist the movement (Fig. 4.30).

Common mistakes:
- In strong subjects the flexion of the knee can not be opposed if the trunk of the examiner is not positioned well over the leg.
- Hyperlordosis can provoke pain in the sacroiliac joints or lumbosacral junction.

Anatomical structures tested:

Muscle function:
- Semimembranosus
- Semitendinosus
- Biceps femoris.

Neural function:

Muscle	Innervation	
	Peripheral	Spinal
Semimembranosus	Sciatic nerve	S1, S2
Semitendinosus	Sciatic nerve	S1, S2
Biceps femoris	Sciatic nerve	S1, S2

Common pathological situations:
- Pain in the thigh is due to a lesion of the hamstrings.
- Weakness is a common sign in first and second root palsies.

Resisted extension of the knee

Positioning. The subject lies prone with the knee flexed to 70°. The examiner stands level with the thigh and leans over the subject. The ipsilateral hand is placed on the distal end of the thigh to stabilize it on the couch. The elbow of the other arm is positioned ventrally around the distal end of the lower leg.

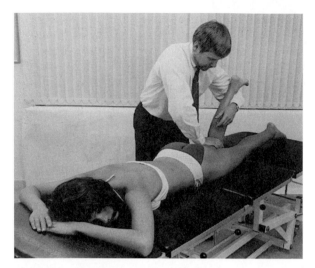

Fig. 4.31 Resisted extension of the knee.

Procedure. Ask the subject to extend the knee, and resist the movement (Fig. 4.31). In order to be able to withstand even the strongest extension, the hand of the supporting arm may grasp the stabilizing arm.

Common mistakes:
- In strong subjects the extension of the knee can not be opposed if the examiner is not leaning in the direction of the subject's head.
- Hyperlordosis may elicit pain from sacroiliac structures or the lumbosacral junction.

Anatomical structures tested:

Muscle function:
- Quadriceps femoris.

Neural function:

Muscle	Innervation	
	Peripheral	Spinal
Quadriceps femoris	Femoralis nerve	L3

Common pathological situations:
- Pain in the thigh is due to a lesion of the quadriceps.
- Weakness is the result of a third lumbar root lesion or a femoralis palsy.

SPECIFIC TESTS

Bilateral passive medial rotation in prone position

Significance

This test is very useful in detecting minor limitations. Since both hips are examined together, even the slightest limitation of medial rotation or a divergence in the end-feel can be detected.

Positioning. The subject lies in the prone position with the knees together and flexed to 90°. The examiner stands at the foot-end of the couch, just distal to the knees, and places both hands against the inner malleoli.

Procedure. Rotate the thighs outwards until the movement comes to a ligamentous stop (Fig. 4.32).

Common mistakes. Care should be taken to keep the buttocks level during the whole procedure.

Common pathological situations:
- A minor limitation may be an early sign of arthritis: this is the first movement to become restricted at the onset of the disease.
- In children either a minor restriction or change in end-feel can be the first sign of Perthes' disease.

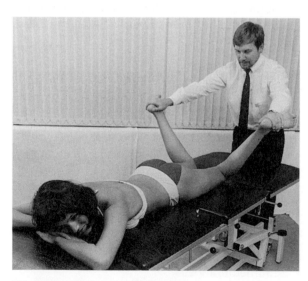

Fig. 4.32 Passive medial rotation.

Adduction in flexion

Significance

This provocation test may be used to compress a painful structure in the groin (psoas bursa or tendon of rectus femoris). However, it should be interpreted with utmost care because other elements such as veins and lymph nodes can also be compressed. This test also stretches several posterior structures (capsule of the hip joint, gluteal muscles and bursae and the sacroiliac joint).

Positioning. The subject lies supine with the hip flexed to a right angle. The examiner stands level with the hip and places one hand on the lateral side of the knee.

Procedure. Force the knee inwards towards the contralateral iliac crest until the movement stops (Fig. 4.33).

Forceful upwards thrust to the heel

Significance

This provocation test may be used to provoke groin pain when an incipient aseptic necrosis of the hip is feared.

Positioning. The subject lies supine with the hip slightly abducted and externally rotated, and the

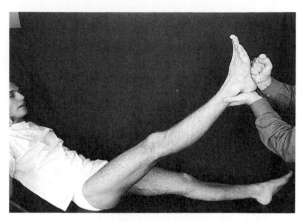

Fig. 4.34   Forceful upwards thrust to the heel.

knee extended. The examiner stands at the foot-end of the couch. One hand carries the heel and lifts the extended leg to 45° (Fig. 4.34).

Procedure. A forceful upwards blow on the heel, axially in the direction of the hip, that provokes groin pain is suggestive of an incipient aseptic necrosis, even in the absence of radiographic signs. Further investigation is mandatory.

Ortolani's test

Significance

This test is used for early detection of congenital dislocation of the hip in babies. During the test a subluxated hip is reduced.

Positioning. The baby lies on its back with the hips flexed to 90° and the knees completely flexed (Fig. 4.35a). The examiner grasps the leg in such a way that the thumb presses on the inner side of the thigh and the ring and middle fingers are on the outer thigh, the tips touching the trochanter.

Procedure (Fig. 4.35b). Abduction is performed. In a subluxated hip, resistance is felt at 45–60°. The moment the resistance is overcome, the femoral head rides over the acetabular edge and reduces. This is felt as a snap.

If the hip displacement is irreducible, a clear limitation of the abduction at the pathological side will be detected.

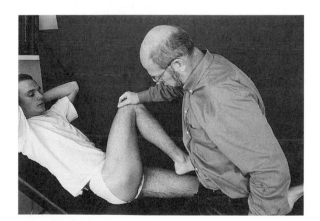

Fig. 4.33   Adduction in flexion.

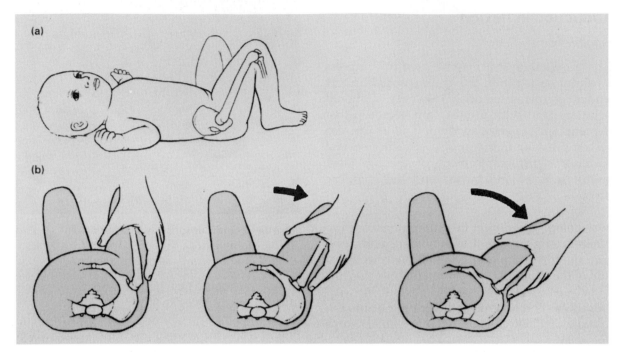

Fig. 4.35 Ortolani's test for congenital dislocation of the hip: (a) position of the baby, (b) reposition of the dislocated hip by abduction.

Barlow's test

Significance

The test is used for early detection of congenital dislocation of the hip in babies. During the test the hip is first subluxated and then replaced.

Positioning. The baby lies on its back, hips flexed to 90° and the knees completely flexed. The examiner grasps the leg in such a way that the thumb presses on the inner side of the thigh and the ring and middle fingers are on the outer thigh, the tips touching the trochanter (Fig. 4.36).

Procedure. If the capsule is elongated, the examiner can press the femoral head outwards and backwards over the acetabular rim. This is indicated by a click. Anterior pressure with the fingertips behind the trochanter can then reduce the hip.

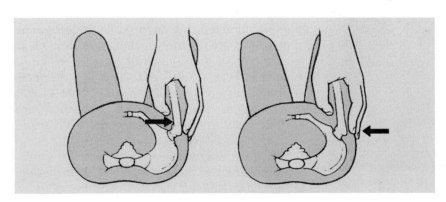

Fig. 4.36 Barlow's test for congenital dislocation of the hip.

5

Knee

SURFACE AND PALPATORY ANATOMY

Bony landmarks (Figs 5.1 and 5.2)

All palpable bony parts of the knee are situated anteriorly. Palpation is performed with the subject in the supine lying position. The knee is either bent to a right angle or fully extended, depending on the palpated structure.

In a flexed position of the knee, the patella can easily be outlined. In this position the large joint line between tibia and femur is situated about two finger-widths below the patellar apex (A).

The inferior part of the medial femoral condyle (B) is easily detectable as a large spherical subcutaneous bony structure that borders the superomedial part of the joint line. The inferior part of the lateral femoral condyle forms the superior border of the lateral joint line (C). Following this condyle in a lateral and posterior direction, the palpating finger encounters the salient lateral epicondyle (D).

The flexed position is also suitable for the palpation of the bony elements of tibia and fibula. The sharp edges of the medial (E) and lateral (F) tibial condyles border the joint line inferiorly and are easy to locate. The tibial tuberosity (G), which is found about two finger-widths below the joint line, is prolonged into the tibial crest (H).

The head of the fibula (I) is easily palpated on a medially rotated leg. Grabbed between thumb and index finger it can be mobilized in an anteroposterior direction (Fig. 5.3).

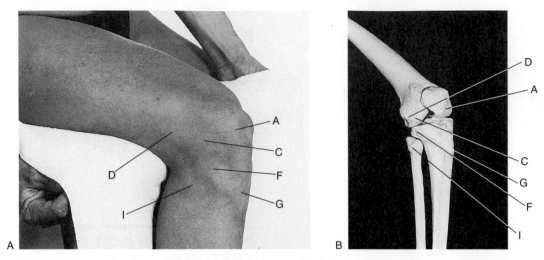

Fig. 5.1 Bony landmarks – anterolateral view: (a) in vivo; (b) skeleton.

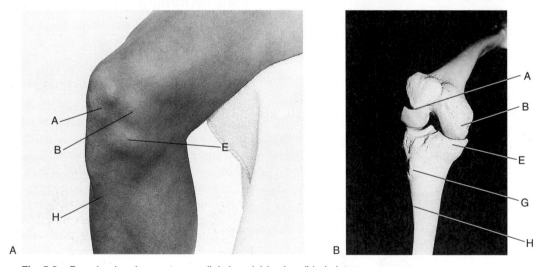

Fig. 5.2 Bony landmarks – anteromedial view: (a) in vivo; (b) skeleton.

The infracondylar tubercle (tubercle of Gerdy), which represents the insertion of the iliotibial tract, is situated on the lateral epicondyle of the tibia, about the width of one thumb below the edge and just in the middle between the tibiofibular joint line and the tibial tuberosity. It is identified as follows: place the thumb of the contralateral hand on the tibial tuberosity and the middle finger on the tibiofibular joint. The index finger, which is slightly more proximal, then touches the tubercle (Fig. 5.4).

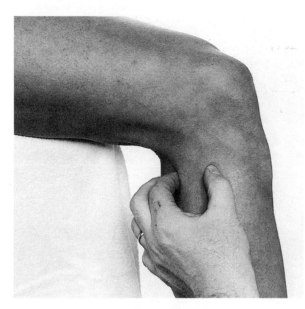

Fig. 5.3 Palpation of the fibular head.

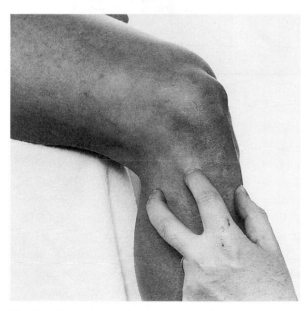

Fig. 5.4 Palpation of the tubercle of Gerdy.

Palpation of the extensor mechanism

This is performed on an extended knee.

First the muscular structures are ascertained. Ask the patient to extend the slightly bent knee and resist the movement.

This movement usually outlines the vastus medialis (A), vastus lateralis (B), rectus femoris (C) and the patellar ligament (D) (Fig. 5.5).

Then the patellar border with its tendinous insertions are palpated. With the hip in flexion and the knee in full extension, the patella can be moved freely upwards and downwards in the patellar groove. Also side gliding and tilting is possible.

The superoposterior border of the bone and the suprapatellar tendon can be palpated after the lower pole of the patella has been pressed posteriorly and upwards by the web of the thumb of the other hand (Figs 5.6 and 5.7).

The medial and lateral edges of the patella together with the quadriceps expansions are palpated in the following way. With the thumb of one hand, the patella is tilted and pushed over

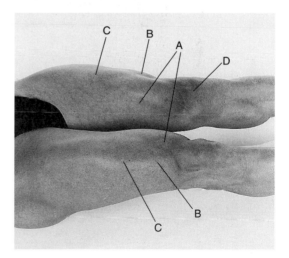

Fig. 5.5 Extensor mechanism of the knee.

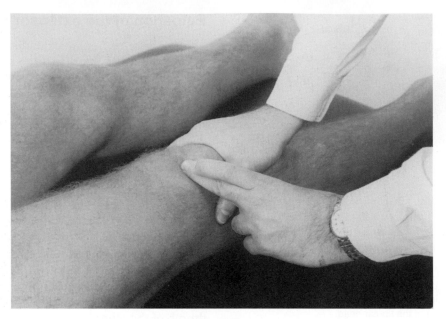

Fig. 5.6 Palpation of the suprapatellar tendon.

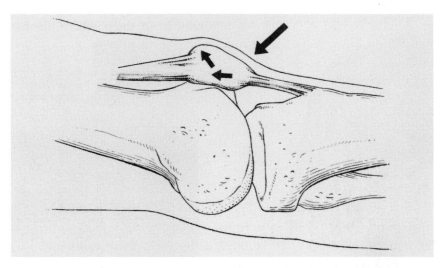

Fig. 5.7 Palpation of the suprapatellar tendon. The patella is tilted (small arrows) by pressing on the inferior pole (large arrow).

to the other side. Place the ring finger of the other hand under the projecting edge and press upwards, squeezing the tendinous fibres against the posterior aspect of the patella (Fig. 5.8).

The inferior pole of the patella and the insertion of the infrapatellar tendon (patellar liga-ment) are palpated in a similar way. Place one hand just above the patella, so that the web of the thumb can exert downwards pressure. This stabilizes the patella and tilts the apex upwards, so it can be palpated with more accuracy (Figs 5.9 and 5.10).

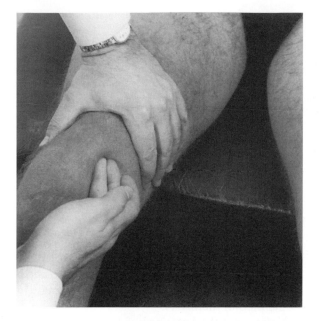

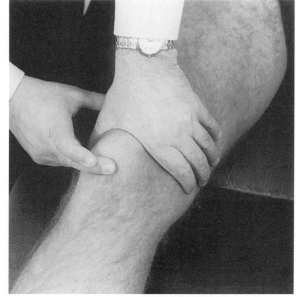

Fig. 5.9 Palpation of the infrapatellar tendon.

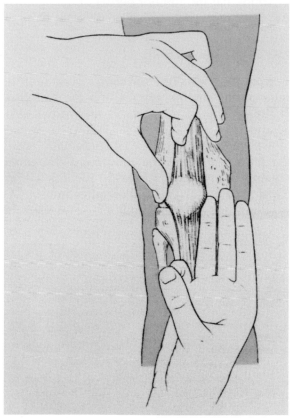

Fig. 5.8 Palpation of the quadriceps extension.

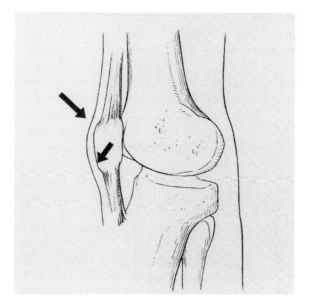

Fig. 5.10 Palpation of the infrapatellar tendon. The patella is pressed distally, which moves the inferior pole upwards (arrows).

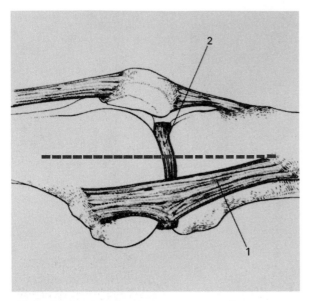

Fig. 5.11 The medial collateral ligament (1) and medial meniscus (2).

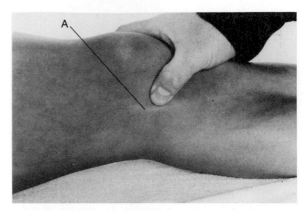

Fig. 5.12 Palpation of the medial collateral ligament.

Palpation of soft tissues at the medial side

Medial collateral ligament

The medial collateral ligament (Fig. 5.11) is a broad, flat and almost triangular band, with a large insertion on the posterosuperior aspect of the medial femoral epicondyle, close to the insertion of the adductor magnus tendon. Its fibres run obliquely, anteriorly and inferiorly, to insert at the medial aspect of the tibia, just behind and slightly under the insertions of the pes anserinus.

The anterior fibres of the ligament are separated from those of the capsule. Therefore the anterior border of the ligament can easily be palpated on an extended knee (Fig. 5.12).

Place the thumb just medially to the patellar tendon and in the intercondylar groove. Palpate the bony borders of the joint line in a posterior direction until the sharp edge of a ligamentous structure is felt to bridge the groove. This is the anterior border of the medial collateral ligament (A). Continue the palpation along the joint line and notice that the bony borders are now covered completely by the dense ligamentous structure. The posterior border of the ligament, however, can not be palpated because the posterior fibres blend intimately with those of the posterior capsule and with the medial and posterior border of the medial meniscus.

Notice that the anterior border of the ligament is situated more posteriorly than is usually thought.

Pes anserinus

The pes anserinus (the common insertion of the semitendinosus, the gracilis and the sartorius) is situated under and behind the medial tibial condyle.

Ask the patient to flex and internally rotate the knee and resist the movement. The three tendinous structures are easily identified from distal to proximal (Fig. 5.13): semitendinosus (A); gracilis (B); and sartorius (C).

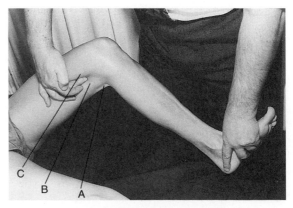

Fig. 5.13 Palpation of the medial tendinous structures.

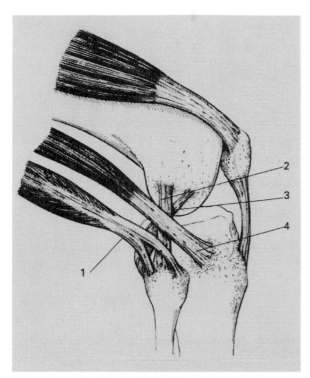

Fig. 5.14 Lateral view of the knee, showing the relations between the lateral muscles and ligaments: 1, biceps femoris; 2, lateral collateral ligament; 3, popliteus; 4, iliotibial tract.

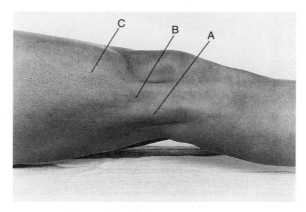

Fig. 5.15 Palpation of the lateral tendinous structures.

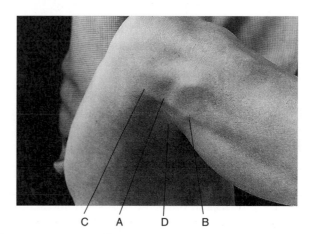

Fig. 5.16 Palpation of the lateral collateral ligament.

Palpation of soft tissues at the lateral side

The lateral side of the knee forms a crossing point of different tendons and ligaments (Fig. 5.14).

The head of the fibula is identified first. A resisted flexion and/or lateral rotation brings the tendon of the biceps femoris (Fig. 5.15, A) into prominence. The tendon inserts at the top and the posterior aspect of the fibular head in two straps, one in front and one behind the insertion of the lateral collateral ligament.

The flexion movement usually also reveals the iliotibial tract (B) which is recognized as a horizontal flat band between biceps and vastus lateralis (C).

The lateral collateral ligament (Fig. 5.16, A) is palpated in the following way. Place the palpating finger on the top of the fibular head (B). Move the leg outwards, meanwhile keeping the foot on the couch (abduction and lateral rotation in the hip). This movement brings the ligament under tension. It is palpated as a tough round structure that runs from the head of the fibula to the lateral femoral epicondyle (C). In this position the ligament makes an 80° angle with the biceps femoris tendon (D).

The intra-articular origin of the popliteus tendon at the lateral condyle is identified as follows.

The knee is still in a flexed position (Fig. 5.17). Identify the lateral border of the patella. The sharp edge of the lateral epicondyle (A) is easily found about one finger-width below the lateral border. Anteriorly a second bony projection is identified as the lateral condyle (B). The groove

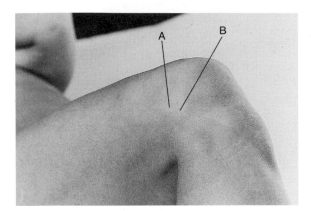

Fig. 5.17 Palpation of the popliteus tendon.

in between these bony structures forms the area from which the tendon emerges. The latter runs intra-articularly and deep to the lateral collateral ligament to continue in the muscle belly that lies deeply in the popliteal fossa under the lateral gastrocnemius and the plantaris muscles.

Palpation of the popliteal fossa

The borders of the lozenge-shaped popliteal fossa (Fig. 5.18) are formed by the gastrocnemii, the biceps femoris and the semitendinosus and semi-membranosus muscles. The bottom is formed by the posterior capsule and the popliteus muscle. The popliteal fossa is covered by a fascia.

The lozenge is vertically crossed (from lateral to medial) by: the tibial nerve, popliteal vein and popliteal artery. The common peroneal nerve descends along the inner border of the biceps.

Palpation is performed with the subject in the prone-lying position. The knee is slightly bent to release the posterior fascia. A slight resisted flexion of the knee brings the upper borders of the popliteal fossa into prominence (Fig. 5.19).

Medially the tendon of the semitendinosus (A) is easily identified as a round cord. The semi-membranosus is situated deeper and has a flatter consistency on palpation.

At the lateral side the biceps tendon (B) can also be recognized easily. Its insertion is on the superior and posterior aspect of the fibular head.

The junction between the semimembranosus

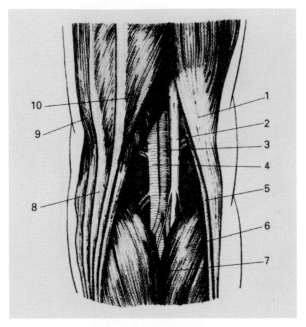

Fig. 5.18 The popliteal fossa: 1, biceps femoris; 2, tibial nerve; 3, popliteal vein; 4, popliteal artery; 5, common peroneal nerve; 6, lateral gastrocnemius; 7, medial gastrocnemius; 8, semimembranosus; 9, gracilis; 10, semitendinosus.

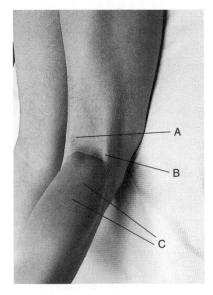

Fig. 5.19 The popliteal fossa in vivo.

and the biceps forms the superior angle of the fossa.

The inferior borders, which are shorter than

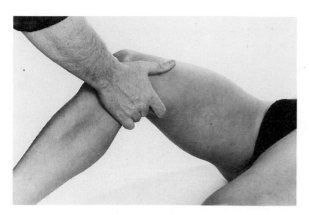

Fig. 5.20 Palpation of the popliteal fossa.

the superior ones, are formed by both gastrocnemii (C). Their junction constitutes the inferior angle of the lozenge. The palpation is facilitated by a resisted plantiflexion of the foot.

The posterior aspects of medial and lateral femoral condyles can be palpated just under the gastrocnemii, the insertion of which is more proximally on the condyles.

The tibial nerve is located in the centre of the lozenge and divides it in two. The tibial vein and the tibial artery are located medial to it.

Nerve and artery can be palpated as follows. The patient is in the supine position, the knee bent to a right angle and the foot flat on the couch. The examiner sits on the couch, next to the knee, and palpates the fossa from the medial aspect with the ipsilateral hand (Fig. 5.20). The nerve is felt as a hard and round structure in the centre of the lozenge, near the upper angle.

To palpate the pulsations of the artery, the fingers must be plunged deeper and more medially.

FUNCTIONAL EXAMINATION OF THE KNEE

Introduction/general remarks

The knee is the largest and most complex joint of the human body. Because it is situated at the ends of two long lever arms it is very well suited to clinical testing. Furthermore, the joint is relatively uncovered by muscles which facilitates palpation of most structures, intra-articular structures excluded.

One should warn against too many different tests. It is important to realize that the quality of a clinical examination does not depend on the number of tests performed but on the accuracy of performance of the most important tests.

Diagnosis of a particular lesion also does not rely on the presence of one pathognomonic test but on the complete clinical picture (the sum of positive and negative answers after the performance of a set of important standardized tests). For instance, none of the so-called pathognomonic meniscus tests has a high positive predicting value (between 21 and 50%) which means that in more than half of the subjects with a positive meniscus test, no meniscal lesion is found on arthroscopy. Also, the presence of a positive instability test has only value if it is interpreted in relation to the rest of the clinical evaluation.

PASSIVE TESTS
Passive flexion

Positioning. The subject lies in the supine position with extended legs. The examiner stands level with the subject's knee. One hand grasps the distal part of the leg, just proximal to the malleoli; the other hand grasps the knee at the medial femoral condyle.

Procedure. Move the extended leg upwards until the knee can be flexed with a simultaneous movement of both hands. Once the flexion has begun, the distal hand continues the movement while the proximal hand just stabilizes the femur in a sagittal plane but allows hip flexion (Fig. 5.21).

Common mistakes. None.

Normal functional anatomy:
- *Range:* 170°
- *End-feel:* soft tissue approximation
- *Limiting structures:* approximation of calf muscles and hamstrings.

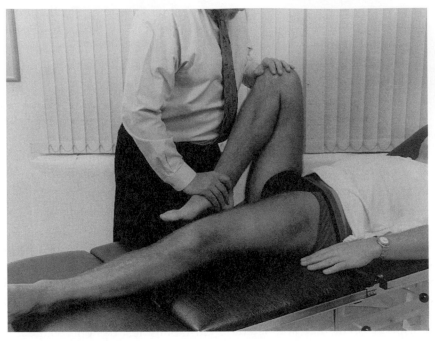

Fig. 5.21   Passive flexion.

Common pathological situations. Numerous conditions lead to limitation in flexion of the knee: capsular lesions, ligamentous adhesions, internal derangement and extra-articular conditions. Diagnosis depends on the pattern that emerges after the completion of the other tests and on the end-feel. A spastic end-feel is typical for acute arthritis or haemarthrosis; a hard end-feel is suggestive of arthrosis, a springy block indicates internal derangement and a soft ligamentous end-feel may be caused by ligamentous adhesions.

Passive extension

Positioning. The subject lies in the supine position with the legs extended. The examiner stands level with the subject's knee. One hand grasps the lower leg at the heel, while the other carries the knee from the lateral side with the thumb on the tibial tuberosity.

Procedure. Move the leg upwards. Perform a quick and short extension movement by a simul-

taneous upwards movement of the heel and a downwards pressure on the tibia (Fig. 5.22).

Common mistakes. The end-feel is not evaluated because the movement is not performed penetratingly enough.

Normal functional anatomy:
- *Range:* 0° (some extension in recurvatum may be possible)
- *End-feel:* hard ligamentous, almost bony
- *Limiting structures:*
    - posterior capsule
    - posterior cruciate ligament
    - anterior cruciate ligament.

Common pathological situations:
- Perception of the end-feel on passive extension is extremely important in clinical diagnosis of knee joint lesions.
- Limited extension with a spastic end-feel in combination with more limitation of flexion indicates an acute arthritis.

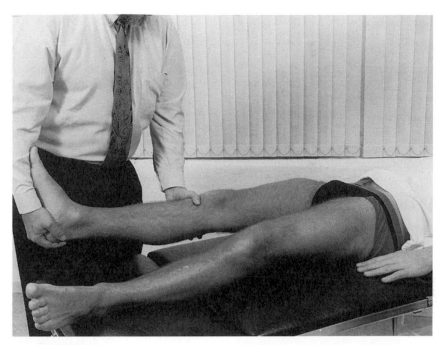

Fig. 5.22 Passive extension.

- Painless and slight limitation with crepitus is typical for arthrosis.
- 10–30° of limitation with a springy block is evidence of a displaced meniscus.
- Pain at the end of range with a more or less normal end-feel is often seen in combination with a small ligamentous problem.

Passive lateral rotation

Positioning. The subject lies in the supine position with the knee flexed to a right angle and the heel resting on the couch. The examiner stands level with the subject's knee. One hand grasps the forefoot at the inner side and presses it upwards in dorsiflexion. Place the other shoulder against the knee, the arm under the lower leg, and the hand under the heel.

Procedure. Perform a lateral rotation by using the foot as a lever; the supporting arm only stabilizes (Fig. 5.23).

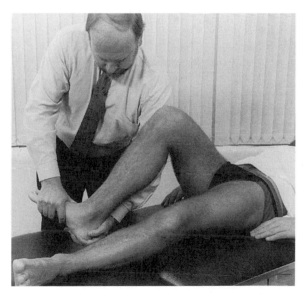

Fig. 5.23 Passive lateral rotation.

Common mistakes. Dorsiflexion in the ankle is lost.

Normal functional anatomy:
- *Range:* 45°
- *End-feel:* elastic ligamentous
- *Limiting structures:*
  - medial meniscotibial (coronary) ligament
  - posterior fibres of medial collateral ligament
  - popliteus muscle.

Passive lateral rotation in prone position

The subject lies in the prone position with both knees flexed to a right angle. The examiner encircles both heels and performs a bilateral external rotation (Fig. 5.24). The range of movement is assessed by the twisted position of the feet.

This test may be decisive in comparing the range of external rotation.

Common pathological situations:
- Pain at the inner side of the knee may indicate a lesion of the medial collateral ligament or the medial coronary ligament.
- Pain at the lateral side suggests a lesion of the popliteus tendon.
- Limitation of the movement is typical for ligamentous adhesions of the medial collateral ligament.
- Increased range of movement in the prone position results from a laxity of the ligamentous structures of the medial compartment and of the anterior cruciate ligament.

Passive medial rotation

Positioning. The subject lies in the supine position with the knee and hip flexed to right angles. The examiner stands level with the subject's knee. One forearm carries the lower leg. The other hand grasps the calcaneus from the lateral side. Both hands clasp tightly under the heel which is forced into dorsiflexion.

Procedure. A combined movement of both wrists turns the lower leg into medial rotation (Fig. 5.25).

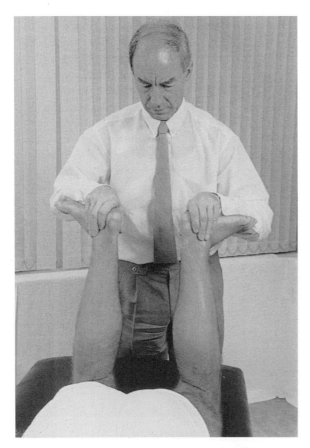

Fig. 5.24 Passive lateral rotation in prone position.

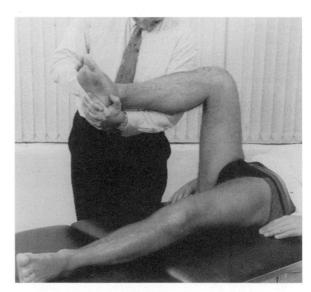

Fig. 5.25 Passive medial rotation.

Common mistakes. The hands are placed too distally on the foot. In order to protect the lateral ligaments, it is important to exert the pressure at the ankle, and not beyond the calcaneocuboid joint line.

Normal functional anatomy:
- *Range:* 30°
- *End-feel:* elastic ligamentous
- *Limiting structures:*
  - lateral meniscotibial (coronary) ligament
  - cruciate ligaments
  - lateral capsular ligaments.

Passive medial rotation in prone position

The subject lies in the prone position with both knees flexed to a right angle. The examiner encircles both heels and performs a bilateral medial rotation. The range of movement is assessed by the twisted position of the feet.

This test compares the range of internal rotation.

Common pathological situations:
- Lateral pain usually indicates a lesion of the lateral coronary ligament.
- An increased range of movement in the prone position is indicative of laxity of the anterior and posterior cruciate ligaments and of the dorsolateral part of the joint capsule.

Valgus strain

Positioning. The subject lies in the supine position with the knees extended. The examiner stands level with the subject's knee. One hand grasps the lower leg from the medial side just proximal to the malleolus. The other hand is supinated and placed at the lateral femoral condyle.

Procedure. Lift the extended leg and apply strong valgus pressure with the distal hand. Counterpressure is maintained at the lateral femoral condyle (Fig. 5.26).

Common mistakes. None.

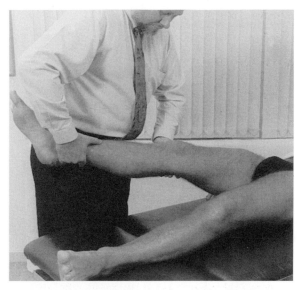

Fig. 5.26 Valgus strain.

Normal functional anatomy:
- *Range:* no movement is possible in a normal knee
- *End-feel:* ligamentous
- *Limiting structures:*
  - medial ligamentous complex
  - cruciate ligaments
  - posterior oblique ligament.

Variation of the valgus test

The test can be repeated with the knee in slight flexion (20–30°). Here the thigh rests on the couch and the lower leg hangs over the edge. Positioning of the hands is the same (Fig. 5.27), as is the procedure.

In this position the cruciate ligaments no longer hold both joint surfaces in firm apposition; therefore some movement can be elicited and more stress is put on the medial ligamentous complex.

Common pathological situations:
- Medial pain during valgus stress is typical for a sprained medial collateral ligament. The test can also be positive in internal derangement of the knee and in medial collateral ligament bursitis.

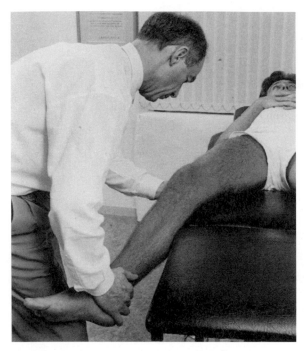

Fig. 5.27   Valgus stress test in 30° of flexion.

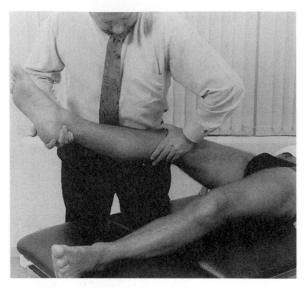

Fig. 5.28   Varus strain.

- Increased range in 30° of flexion is typical for a rupture of the medial compartment ligaments.
- If valgus stress in full extension also shows an increased range, the posterior cruciate ligament is probably torn as well.

Varus strain

Positioning. The subject lies in the supine position with the knees extended. The examiner stands level with the subject's knee. The ipsilateral hand grasps the lower leg from the lateral side, just proximal to the lateral malleolus. The other hand is pronated and placed at the medial femoral condyle.

Procedure. Lift the extended leg and apply strong varus pressure with the distal hand. Counterpressure is maintained at the medial femoral condyle (Fig. 5.28).

Common mistakes. The knee is not fully extended during the procedure.

Normal functional anatomy:
- *Range*: in a normal knee no perceptible movement is possible
- *End-feel*: hard ligamentous
- *Limiting structures*:
  – lateral collateral ligament
  – arcuate ligament
  – posterior cruciate ligament.

Variation of the varus test

The test can be repeated with the knee in slight flexion (20–30°). Here the thigh rests on the couch and the lower leg hangs over the edge. The examiner stands distal to the foot. Again, the lower hand provokes a varus strain while the hand at the knee stabilizes (Fig. 5.29).

In this position the cruciate ligaments no longer hold both joint surfaces in firm apposition; therefore some movement is possible and more stress is put on the lateral ligamentous complex.

Common pathological situations:
- Lateral pain during varus stress inculpates the lateral collateral ligament; medial pain may accompany an impacted loose body or impacted medial meniscus.

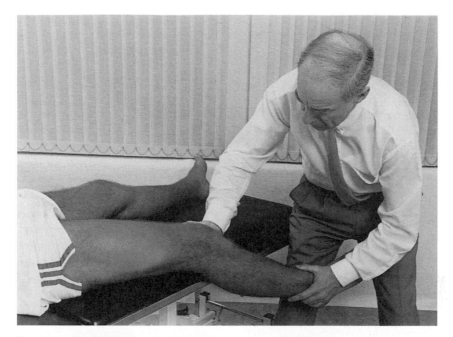

Fig. 5.29   Varus stress test in 30° of flexion.

- Increased range in 30° of flexion is typical for a rupture of the lateral collateral ligament.
- If varus stress in full extension also shows an increased range, the posterior cruciate ligament is probably torn as well.

Anterior drawer test

Positioning. The subject lies in the supine position with the knee flexed to a right angle, and the heel resting on the couch. The examiner sits on the foot of the subject. One hand is on the anterior aspect of the knee: apex patellae in the palm of the hand, thenar and hypothenar making contact with the femoral condyles. The other hand is at the back of the upper tibia.

Procedure. Draw the tibia forwards with the posterior hand and add a strong jerk when the movement comes to a stop. The hand on the patella stabilizes the thigh (Fig. 5.30).

Common mistakes. None.

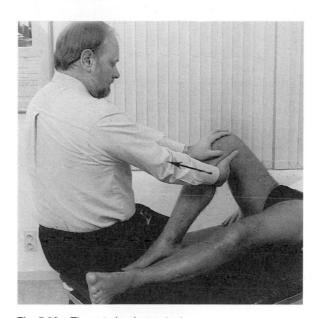

Fig. 5.30   The anterior drawer test.

Normal functional anatomy:
- *Range*: in a normal joint the tibia shifts over only a few millimetres
- *End-feel*: hard ligamentous
- *Limiting structures*: anterior cruciate ligament.

Common pathological situations:

- Pain is indicative of a small lesion of the anterior cruciate ligament.
- Increase in range is seen in ruptures of the anterior cruciate ligament and/or the posterior capsule.

Anterior drawer test in external rotation

Positioning. The subject is positioned as for the previous test. The lower leg and foot are externally rotated as far as is comfortably possible. The examiner places both hands around the upper part of the tibia with the index fingers on the hamstring tendons and the thumbs at the anterior border of the joint (Fig. 5.31).

Procedure. Draw the upper part of the tibia forwards and add a strong jerk at the end of the movement.

Normal findings. The range of movement in external rotation is slightly superior to the movement in a neutral position.

Common pathological situations. A marked increase in range is indicative of anteromedial rotatory instability (ruptures of the anterior cruciate ligament, the posteromedial capsule and the medial collateral ligament).

Anterior drawer test in internal rotation

Positioning. The subject is positioned as for the previous test. The lower leg and foot are internally rotated as far as is comfortably possible. The examiner places both hands around the upper part of the tibia with the index fingers on the hamstring tendons and the thumbs at the the anterior border of the joint (Fig. 5.32).

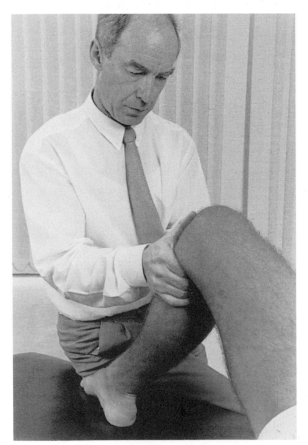

Fig. 5.31   Anterior drawer test in external rotation.

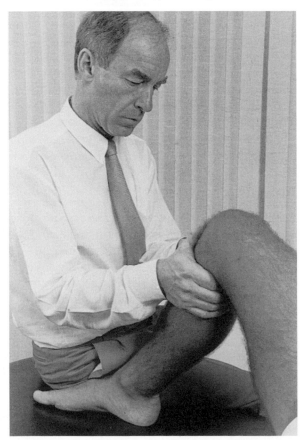

Fig. 5.32   Anterior drawer test in internal rotation.

Procedure. Draw the upper part of the tibia forwards and add a strong jerk at the end of range.

Common pathological situations. Internal rotation tightens the intact posterior cruciate ligament which prevents any movement.

Variation: anterior drawer in 20° of flexion (Lachman test)

Positioning. The subject lies in the supine position with the legs extended. The examiner stands level with the knee. One hand grasps the proximal tibia from the medial side, the fingers in the popliteal fossa and the thumb at the tibial tuberosity. The other hand holds the distal femur from the lateral side, the thumb just proximal to the patella.

Procedure. Bring the knee into about 20° of flexion and, using both hands, displace the proximal tibia anteriorly (Fig. 5.33).

Common mistakes. None.

Normal functional anatomy:
- *Range*: in a normal knee only a small amplitude of anterior glide (less than 5 mm) is obtainable
- *End-feel*: ligamentous
- *Limiting structures*: anterior cruciate ligament.

Common pathological situations. This test is preferred to detect ruptures of the anterior cruciate ligament.

Posterior drawer test

Positioning. The subject lies in the supine position with the knee flexed to a right angle, and the heel resting on the couch. The examiner sits on the foot of the subject. The heel of one hand is placed on the tibial tuberosity and the other hand is placed at the back of the upper tibia.

Procedure. Push the tibia backwards with a strong jerk of the anterior hand (Fig. 5.34). The posterior hand in the popliteal fossa discloses any eventual movement.

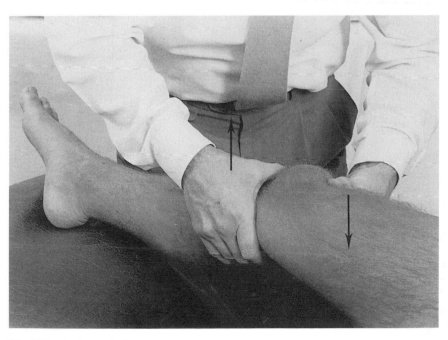

Fig. 5.33 Lachman test.

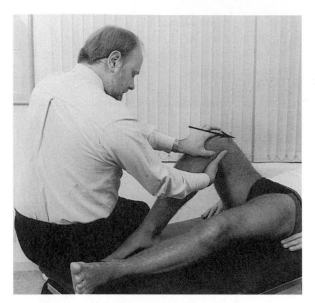

Fig. 5.34 The posterior drawer test.

Common mistakes. None.

Normal functional anatomy:
- *Range*: no movement can be provoked in a normal knee

- *End-feel*: hard ligamentous
- *Limiting structures*: posterior cruciate ligament.

Common pathological situations:
- Pain is indicative of a small lesion of the posterior cruciate ligament.
- Increase in range is seen in ruptures of the posterior cruciate ligament and / or the arcuate complex.

ISOMETRIC CONTRACTIONS
Resisted extension

Positioning. The subject lies in the supine position with the knee slightly bent. The examiner stands level with the knee. One forearm is placed under the knee with the hand resting on the other knee, proximal to the patella. The other hand is on the distal end of the leg just proximal to the malleoli.

Procedure. The subject is asked to extend the knee and to maintain extension while the examiner pushes the lower leg down towards the couch (Fig. 5.35).

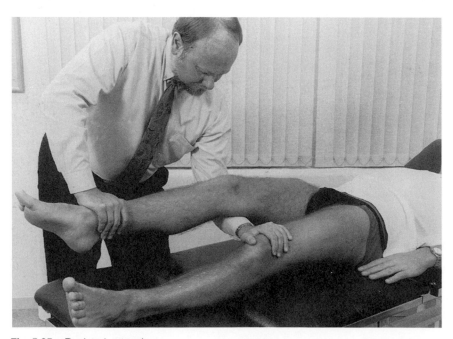

Fig. 5.35 Resisted extension.

Common mistakes. None.

Anatomical structures tested:

Muscle function:
- Quadriceps femoris
- Tensor fasciae latae.

Neural function:

Muscle	Innervation	
	Peripheral	Spinal
Quadriceps femoris	Femoralis	L3
Tensor fasciae latae	Superior gluteal	L5

Resisted flexion

Positioning. The subject lies in the supine position with the hip and knee bent to right angles. The examiner stands level with the foot of the subject. Both hands support the heel (Fig. 5.36).

Procedure. The subject is asked to move the heel downwards while the examiner applies strong counterpressure.

Common mistakes. None.

Anatomical structures tested:

Muscle function:
- Semimembranosus
- Semitendinosus
- Biceps femoris
- Popliteus
- Gastrocnemii
- Plantaris
- Gracilis
- Sartorius
- Tensor fasciae latae.

Indirect traction on inert structures:
- Proximal tibiofibular joint
- Posterior cruciate ligament
- Posterior horn of the medial meniscus.

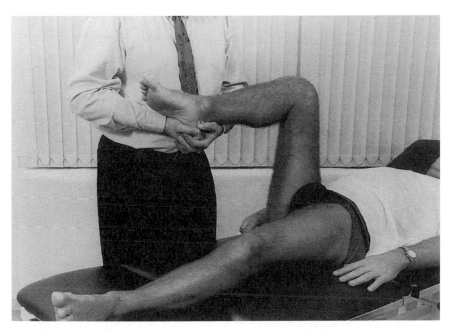

Fig. 5.36 Resisted flexion.

Neural function:

Muscle	Innervation	
	Peripheral	Spinal
Semimembranosus	Sciatic nerve	S1, S2
Semitendinosus	Sciatic nerve	S1, S2
Biceps femoris	Sciatic nerve	S1, S2
Gracilis	Obturator	L2, L3, L4
Sartorius	Femoral	L2, L3
Tensor fasciae latae	Superior gluteal	L5
Popliteus	Tibial	L4, L5, S1
Gastrocnemii	Tibial	S1, S2
Plantaris	Tibial	S1, S2

Resisted medial rotation

Positioning. The subject sits with the lower legs pendent. The examiner squats in front of the knee. The ipsilateral hand encircles the heel from the lateral side. The contralateral hand is placed against the medial aspect of the forefoot and holds the foot in dorsiflexion (Fig. 5.37).

Procedure. The subject is asked to turn the foot inwards while the examiner applies strong counter-pressure with both hands.

Common mistakes. Not enough dorsiflexion makes the subject execute an inversion of the foot.

Anatomical structures tested:

Muscle function:
- Semimembranosus
- Semitendinosus
- Gracilis
- Sartorius
- Popliteus.

Indirect traction on inert structures:
- Posterior horn of the medial meniscus.

Neural function:

Muscle	Innervation	
	Peripheral	Spinal
Semimembranosus	Sciatic nerve	S1, S2
Semitendinosus	Sciatic nerve	S1, S2
Gracilis	Obturator	L2, L3, L4
Sartorius	Femoral	L2, L3
Popliteus	Tibial	(L4), L5, S1

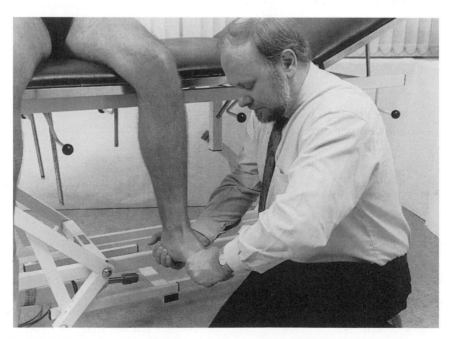

Fig. 5.37   Resisted medial rotation.

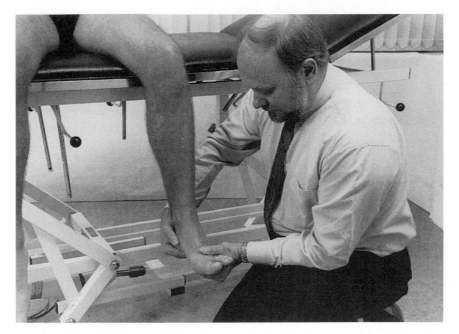

Fig. 5.38 Resisted lateral rotation.

Resisted lateral rotation

Positioning. The subject sits with the lower legs pendent. The examiner squats in front of the knee. The ipsilateral hand is placed against the lateral aspect of the forefoot and maintains dorsiflexion. The contralateral hand encircles the heel from the medial side (Fig. 5.38).

Procedure. The patient is asked to turn the foot outwards while the examiner applies strong counter-pressure.

Common mistakes. If dorsiflexion is not maintained, the subject will execute an eversion of the foot.

Anatomical structures tested:

Muscle function:
- Biceps femoris
- Tensor fasciae latae.

Indirect traction on inert structures:
- Proximal tibiofibular joint

Neural function:

Muscle	Innervation	
	Peripheral	Spinal
Biceps femoris	Sciatic nerve	S1, S2
Tensor fasciae latae	Superior gluteal	L5

SPECIFIC TESTS

Medial shearing

Significance

This test is used to detect internal derangement at the inner side of the knee. Pain on jerk is suggestive for a minor lesion at the tibial insertion of the anterior cruciate ligament.

Positioning. The subject lies in the supine position with the knee flexed to a right angle, and the heel resting on the couch. The examiner sits at the foot-end of the couch. The heel of the ipsilateral hand is placed at the medial femoral condyle. The heel of the contralateral hand is at the lateral tibial condyle. The fingers of both hands are interlocked.

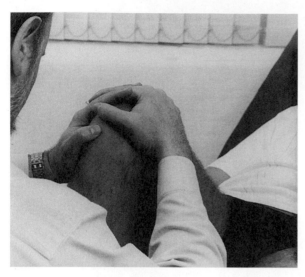

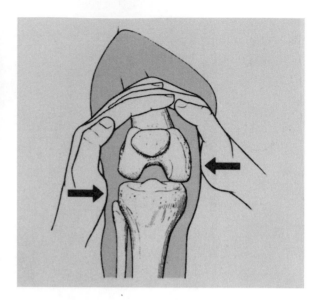

Fig. 5.39 Medial shearing strain.

Procedure Apply a strong shearing strain that forces the tibia medially on the femur (Fig. 5.39).

Common mistakes:
- The hands are not high enough on the femur or low enough on the tibia respectively.
- The contralateral hand presses against the fibular head instead of the lateral tibial condyle, provoking a painful compression of the upper tibiofibular joint.

Normal functional anatomy:
- *Range*: Virtually no movement can be elicited in a normal knee
- *End-feel*: hard ligamentous
- *Limiting structures*:
  - articular surfaces
  - intercondylar spines of the tibia
  - menisci
  - anterior cruciate ligament.

Lateral shearing

Significance

This test is used to detect internal derangement at the outer side of the knee.

Positioning. The subject lies in the supine position, with the knee flexed to a right angle and the heel resting on the couch. The examiner sits opposite the subject at the foot-end of the couch. The heel of the ipsilateral hand is placed at the medial tibial condyle. The heel of the contralateral hand is placed at the lateral femoral condyle. The fingers of both hands are interlocked.

Procedure. Apply a strong shearing strain that forces the tibia laterally on the femur (Fig. 5.40).

Common mistakes. The hands are not high enough on the femur or low enough on the tibia respectively.

Normal functional anatomy:
- *Range*: no movement can be elicited in a normal knee
- *End-feel*: hard ligamentous
- *Limiting structures*:
  - articular surfaces
  - intercondylar spines of the tibia
  - menisci
  - posterior cruciate ligament.

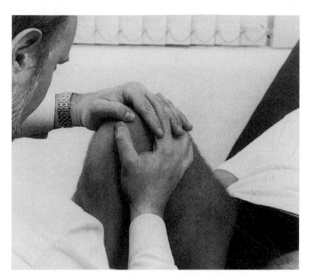

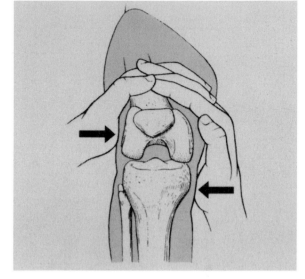

Fig. 5.40 Lateral shearing strain.

Provocation tests for meniscal tears

Significance

These tests are used to detect, by demonstration of clicks and/or pain, meniscal tears in the absence of actual (sub)luxations. If clicks are detected, it is wise to examine the other limb as well in order to eliminate non-pathological clicks arising from tendons snapping over bony prominences.

Test I

Positioning. The subject lies supine with the knee fully flexed. The examiner holds his index finger and thumb at both sides of the infrapatellar tendon, level with the joint line. The other hand grasps the heel (Fig. 5.41).

Procedure. The leg is rotated quickly to and fro. When clicks are felt at the joint line, a ruptured meniscus should be suspected.

Test II (McMurray test)

Positioning. The subject lies supine with the knee fully flexed (heel to the buttock). The examiner

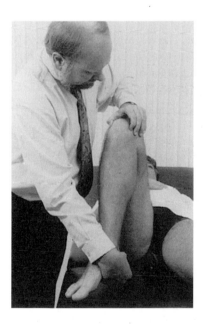

Fig. 5.41 Test to detect clicks during rotation in full flexion.

holds a palpating finger in the joint line at the side to be tested. The other hand grasps the heel and rotates the leg fully (externally to test the medial meniscus, internally for the lateral meniscus).

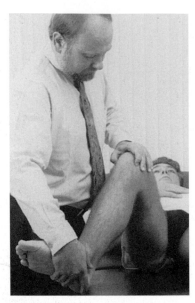

Fig. 5.42 Test to detect a click during extension movement under external rotation.

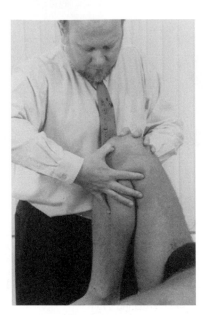

Fig. 5.43 Palpation of a displaced rim.

Procedure. The examiner now slowly extends the knee, while rotation is maintained (Fig. 5.42). As extension proceeds, a click may be felt, usually as the leg approaches the neutral position.

Test III

Positioning. The subject lies supine with the knee fully flexed (heel to the buttock). The examiner passes his flexed thumbtip from above downwards over the joint line at the affected side (Fig. 5.43). This is easier to perform at the medial side than on the lateral.

Procedure. A ruptured meniscus is suspected when it is possible to hook the rim of the meniscus and pull it downwards until it is felt to jump back in place again.

Specific tests for instability

Significance

Most instability can usually be detected by the earlier described passive movements. There are, however, valuable specific tests: the 'jerk' test and 'pivot shift' for anterolateral rotatory insta-

bility and the external rotation–recurvatum test for posterolateral rotatory instability.

Lateral pivot shift (test of MacIntosh)

Positioning. The subject lies supine with the hip flexed to about 30° and slightly medially rotated. The knee is extended. The examiner supports the patient's leg, with one hand at the foot and the other at the knee, the thumb behind the fibular head.

Procedure. The hand at the foot rotates the tibia internally, while the other hand exerts a mild valgus stress at the knee. The examiner flexes the knee gradually, maintaining the internal rotation and valgus stress. In anterolateral rotatory instability the lateral tibial condyle will first subluxate anteriorly and, at approximately 30° of flexion, reduce suddenly backwards. This posterior bouncing is seen and felt both by examiner and subject and indicates a positive test.

The 'jerk' test

Positioning. The subject lies supine with the hip flexed to about 45°, and the knee to 90°. The

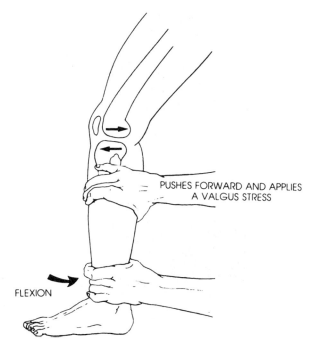

Fig. 5.44 Lateral pivot shift. (From Magee D J 1997 Orthopedic physical assessment, 3rd edn. W B Saunders, Philadelphia.)

PUSHES FORWARD AND APPLIES A VALGUS STRESS

FLEXION

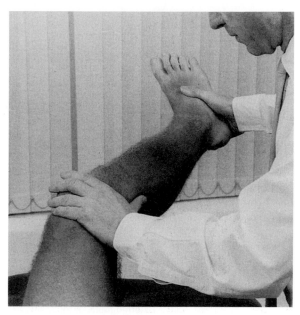

Fig. 5.45 The 'jerk' test.

examiner supports the subject's leg, with one hand at the foot and the other at the knee, the thumb behind the fibular head.

Procedure. The hand at the foot rotates the tibia slightly internally, while the other hand exerts a mild valgus stress at the knee. The examiner extends the knee gradually, maintaining the internal rotation and valgus stress (Fig. 5.45). A positive result is indicated if, on attaining about 30° of flexion, anterior subluxation of the tibia occurs with a sudden movement, which is called a jerk. The forwards shift can be seen and felt by the examiner. At the same moment, the subject will recognize the feeling of instability.

External recurvatum test

Positioning. The subject lies supine with both legs relaxed and extended. The examiner grasps the big toes.

Procedure. Both legs are lifted simultaneously (Fig. 5.46). The amount of external rotation of the

tibial plateau and the degree of recurvatum are observed. In a positive test, unilateral excess of external rotation and recurvatum is seen.

Tests for fluid

Fluid in the knee joint is a sign common to many disorders (traumatic, inflammatory or crystalline). Three tests are commonly used to detect fluid.

Patellar tap

Positioning. The subject lies supine with the knee extended or flexed to discomfort. The examiner stands level with the knee. The web of one hand is on the suprapatellar pouch. The thumb and middle finger of the other hand press at the medial and lateral recessi, just beyond the patellar edges (Fig. 5.47).

Procedure. Manual pressure empties the recessi and moves the fluid between patella and femur. The index finger of the other hand pushes the patella downwards. If fluid is present, one can feel the patella move. When it strikes the femur, a palpable tap is felt followed by an immediate

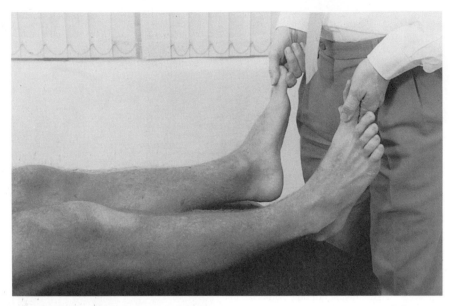

Fig. 5.46 External rotation–recurvatum test.

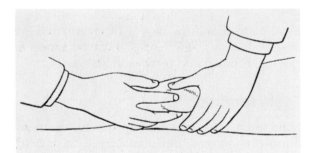

Fig. 5.47 Testing for fluid in the joint by patellar tap.

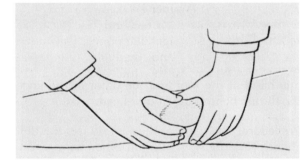

Fig. 5.48 Testing for fluid in the joint by eliciting fluctuation.

upwards movement. This is the sensation of an ice cube pushed downwards in a glass of water: although the patella moves downwards, the pressure of the fluid immediately shifts the bone upwards against the palpating finger.

Remark: when large amounts of fluid are present, the tap of the patella hitting the femur cannot be felt.

Eliciting fluctuation

Positioning. The subject lies in the supine position with the leg extended. The examiner stands level with the knee. He places thumb and index finger of one hand at each side of the knee, just beyond the patella. The interdigital web I–II of the other hand is on the suprapatellar pouch (Fig. 5.48).

Procedure. The examiner squeezes the suprapatellar pouch, pushing all the fluid downwards under the patella, which forces the two fingers of the palpating hand apart.

Visual testing by eliciting fluctuation

Positioning. The subject lies in the supine position with the leg extended.

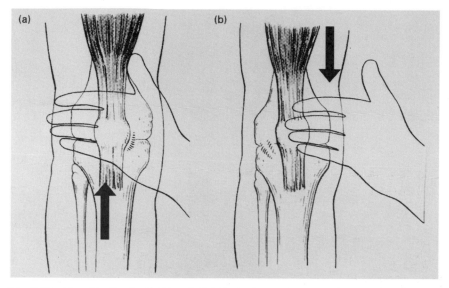

Fig. 5.49 Visual testing for fluid by eliciting fluctuation.

Procedure. The examiner strokes in a sweeping motion with the back of one hand over the lateral recessus and the suprapatellar pouch. This moves the fluid upwards and medially (Fig. 5.49a). In minor effusion, all the fluid is moved to the medial part of the suprapatellar pouch. The lateral recessus is then empty and can be seen as a groove between patella and lateral femoral condyle. Sweeping with the back of the hand over the suprapatellar pouch, and downwards over the medial recessus will now transfer the fluid laterally where a small prominence appears (Fig. 5.49b). This is the most delicate test for effusion in the knee joint, and will even demonstrate 2 or 3 ml of fluid.

Synovial thickening

Synovial thickening is a vital clinical finding. It indicates primary inflammation of the synovia and differentiates this from a secondary synovitis.

Synovial swelling is best detected at the medial and lateral condyles of the femur (Fig. 5.50), about 2 cm posterior to the medial and lateral edges of the patella. Here the capsule lies almost superficially, covered only by skin and subcutaneous

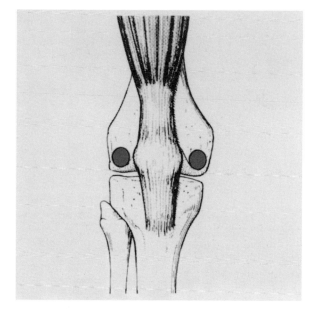

Fig. 5.50 Detection of synovial thickness.

fat. It is palpated by rolling the structures between fingertip and bone. Normally nothing except skin can be felt. In synovial thickening, a dense structure can be felt.

6

Ankle and foot

SURFACE AND PALPATORY ANATOMY

POSTERIOR

Bony landmarks (Figs 6.1 and 6.2)

Calcaneus, medial and lateral malleolus are visible landmarks. The upper surface of the tuber

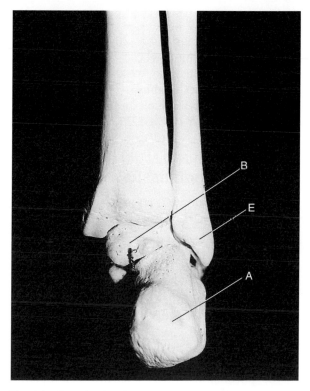

Fig. 6.1   Bony landmarks on skeleton.

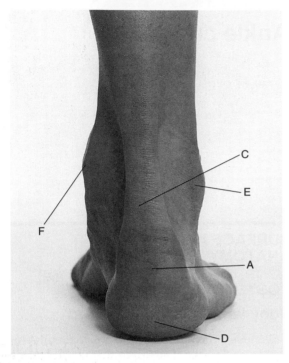

Fig. 6.2 Bony landmarks in vivo.

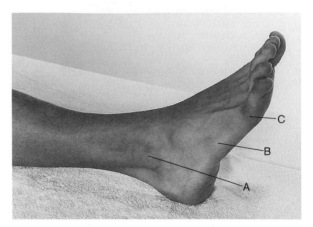

Fig. 6.3 Bony landmarks at the lateral ankle.

calcanei (A) can easily be palpated and forms the basis of the triangle whose legs are formed by the anterior border of the Achilles tendon and the posterior aspect of the tibia.

The posterior border of the talus (B), nipped between tibia and calcaneu, is hardly palpable as a small crest.

Palpation of soft tissue (Figs 6.1 and 6.2)

The Achilles tendon (C) is easily visible and palpable. It inserts at the upper and posterior border of the calcaneus.

The plantar aspect of the calcaneus is covered by a soft heel pad (D). The tip of the lateral malleolus is level with the lateral joint line of the talocalcanean joint. Its inferior border extends about 1 cm further distally than that of the medial malleolus.

The posterior surface of the lateral malleolus (E) carries a sulcus which contains the tendons of the peronei. The peroneus brevis is against the bone with the tendon of the peroneus longus

on top of it. The posterior surface of the medial malleolus (F) also bears a groove in which the tibialis posterior tendon can be palpated (see palpation of medial structures).

LATERAL
Bony landmarks (Fig. 6.3)

The lateral malleolus (A), the base of the fifth metatarsal (B) and the fifth metatarsophalangeal joint (C) constitute the important bony landmarks at the lateral aspect of ankle and foot. From these bony points nearly all palpable lateral structures can be ascertained.

Palpation of the peronei
(Figs 6.4 and 6.5)

About one finger-breadth under and slightly anterior to the lateral malleolus, a bony notch can be palpated: the trochlear process (A). Since this prominence is situated between both peroneal tendons, the palpating finger will be lifted off by the hardening tendons when an eversion movement is performed. The peroneus longus (B) is plantar and the peroneus brevis (C) is dorsal to the trochlear process. The tendon of the peroneus longus can be followed proximally under and behind the malleolus. The tendon of the peroneus brevis is felt to insert on the base of the fifth metatarsal.

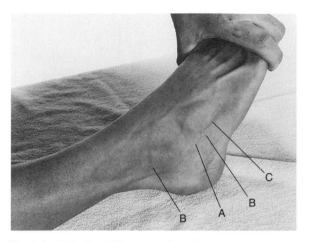

Fig. 6.4   Palpation of the peronei.

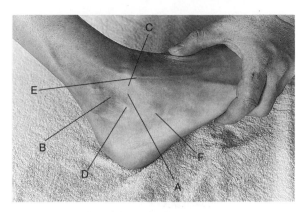

Fig. 6.6   Palpation of the sinus tarsi in vivo.

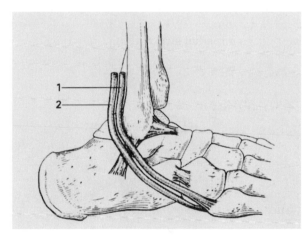

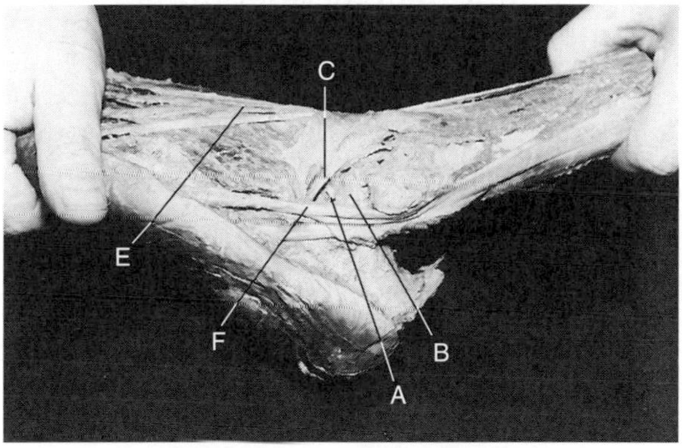

Fig. 6.5   The peroneal tendons: 1, peroneus brevis; 2, peroneus longus.

Fig. 6.7   Palpation of the sinus tarsi.

Palpation of the sinus tarsi
(Figs 6.6 and 6.7)

Starting from the anterior surface of the lateral malleolus and moving anteriorly and medially, the finger falls into a depression – the sinus tarsi (A). If the finger is left in place and the foot is inverted, the depression excavates and its borders can be better ascertained. Just anterior to the malleolus the lateral process of the talus (B) is felt to press against the palpating finger. The neck of the talus (C) is determined as the medial border and the anterior third of the calcaneus (D) as the bottom of the sinus tarsi.

The sinus tarsi is also bordered by tendinous structures: superiorly the long extensors of the toes (E) and inferiorly the peronei (F).

Palpation of the anterior talofibular ligament (Fig. 6.8)

The index finger is laid on the anterior surface of the lateral malleolus. A combined plantar flexion–inversion movement of the ankle makes the lateral process of the talus more prominent. The ligament is felt as a thin, flat and horizontal structure, pressing against the palpating finger.

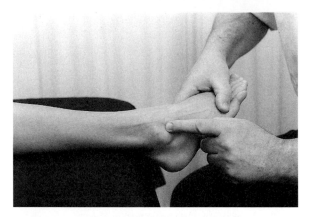

Fig. 6.8 Palpation of the anterior talofibular ligament.

Palpation of the calcaneofibular ligament (Figs 6.9 and 6.10)

One finger is placed just caudal and posterior to the lateral malleolus. The other hand encircles the heel and provokes a varus movement in the subtalar joint. A strong and round structure with a slight posterior inclination is felt to press against the palpating finger (the calcaneofibular ligament (A)).

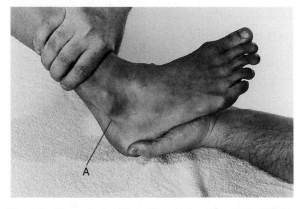

Fig. 6.9 The calcaneofibular ligament can be made visible during a strong varus movement.

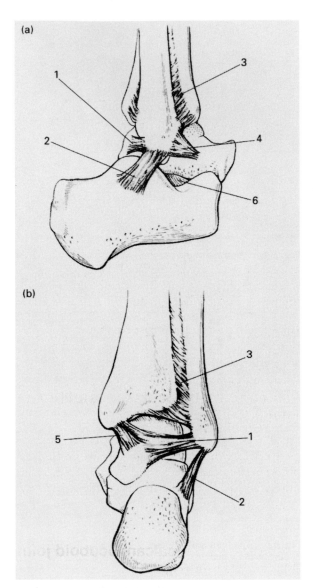

Fig. 6.10 Lateral and posterior ligaments of the ankle (a) lateral view; (b) posterior view: 1, posterior talofibular ligament; 2, calcaneofibular ligament; 3, distal tibiofibular ligament; 4, anterior talofibular ligament; 5, posterior tibiotalar ligament; 6, tarsal canal.

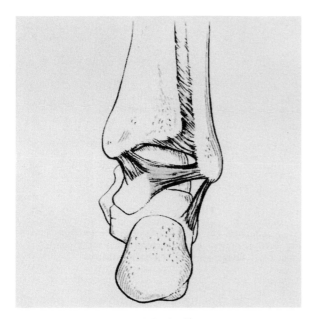

Fig. 6.11   The posterior talofibular ligament.

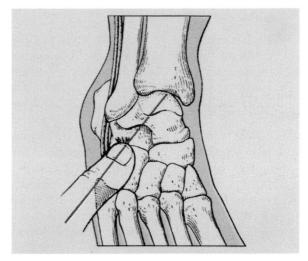

Fig. 6.12   Palpation technique for the calcaneocuboid ligament.

Palpation of the posterior talofibular ligament (Fig. 6.11)

Place the palpating finger deeply behind the lateral malleolus and search for the lateral and posterior aspects of the talus. A dorsiflexion movement in the ankle makes the taut ligament press against the finger.

Palpation of the calcaneocuboid joint and ligaments (Fig. 6.12)

The examiner places the interphalangeal joint of his thumb on the base of the fifth metacarpal bone and aims in the direction of the midpoint between the two malleoli. The tip of the palpating thumb now lies exactly on the lateral calcaneocuboid ligament. In neutral position the joint line can clearly be ascertained. The ligament can be felt when it is brought under tension during supination and adduction of the foot.

Palpation of the cuboid–metatarsal V joint (Fig 6.13)

The base of the fifth metatarsal bone is gripped between the thumb and index of one hand. The cuboid bone (medial to the metatarsal and distal to the already identified calcaneocuboid joint line) is gripped between the thumb and index finger of the other hand. A translation movement discloses easily the joint line between cuboid and fifth metatarsal bone.

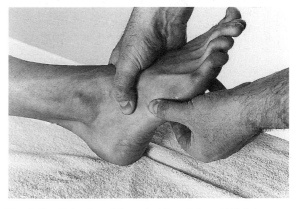

Fig. 6.13   Palpation of the cuboid–metatarsal V joint.

MEDIAL

The medial malleolus, the sustentaculum tali, the tuberosity of the scaphoid and the base of the first metatarsal bone constitute the important bony landmarks at the medial aspect of the ankle and foot. The medial malleolus (Fig. 6.14, A) is felt with ease. The sustentaculum tali (B) is found about 2 cm below the tip of the medial malleolus. This bony prominence is better palpable if the calcaneus is pushed into a valgus position.

The tuberosity of the scaphoid bone (Fig. 6.15, A) is found as follows. Ask for and resist an inversion movement of the foot which brings the strong tibialis posterior and anterior tendons into

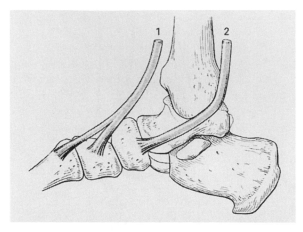

Fig. 6.16   Tendons and insertions of the main invertor muscles: 1, tibialis anterior; 2, tibialis posterior.

prominence. The insertion of the tibialis posterior tendon (B) is on the tuberosity (Fig. 6.16).

The tibialis anterior tendon (C) is followed along the medial border of the foot where it is felt to insert on a bony prominence, the tubercle of the first metatarsal base (D). This point is the midpoint of the medial border of the foot.

The talar head can be palpated at the midpoint of a line joining the tip of the malleolus to the tuberosity of the scaphoid bone (Fig. 6.17). The talonavicular joint becomes more apparent during an adduction movement in the midfoot.

The thick structures that are palpable just around the inferior border of the medial malleolus constitute the different layers of the deltoid liga-

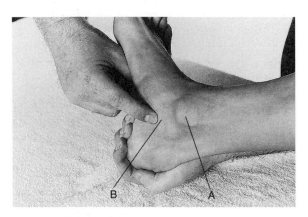

Fig. 6.14   Palpation of the medial malleolus and the sustentaculum tali.

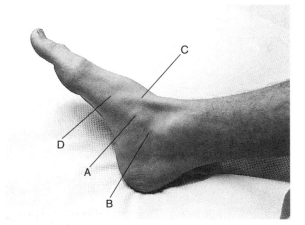

Fig. 6.15   Visualization of medial structures.

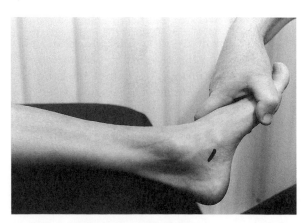

Fig. 6.17   Visualization of the talar head.

ment. They become more obvious when a varus movement is performed.

The ligament that connects the sustentaculum tali with the inferior surface of the navicular bone is the inferior calcaneonavicular ligament (spring ligament) (Fig. 6.18 and Fig. 6.19, B). It is best palpated on a passively everted foot. Since the insertion on the navicular bone is close to that of the tibialis posterior tendon (A), both structures will constitute a V that can be felt during a resisted inversion of the foot.

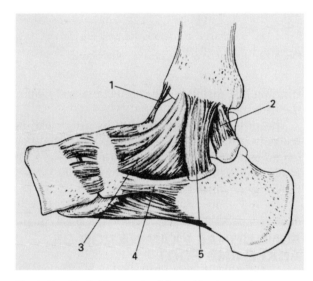

Fig. 6.18 Medial ligaments of the ankle: 1, anterior tibiotalar ligament; 2, posterior tibiotalar ligament; 3, tibionavicular ligament; 4, inferior calcaneonavicular ligament; 5, tibiocalcanear ligament.

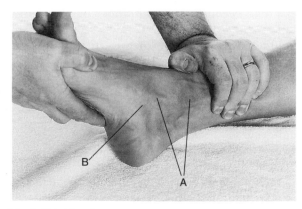

Fig. 6.19 Visualization of the spring ligament.

The following longitudinal structures can be palpated along the posterior aspect of the medial malleolus from anterior to posterior successively: the tibialis posterior and flexor digitorum longus tendons, the posterior tibial artery and the flexor hallucis longus tendon (Fig. 6.20a).

The tibialis posterior tendon remains in contact with the bone of the malleolus and becomes prominent during an inversion movement (Fig. 6.19). The tendon of the flexor digitorum longus is difficult to palpate and is situated more laterally and dorsally. Behind this tendon the pulse of the posterior tibial artery can be felt.

The flexor hallucis longus tendon (Fig. 6.20b and Fig. 6.21, A) is identified as follows. Place the palpating finger between the medial malleolus and the anterior aspect of the Achilles tendon. Bring the foot into dorsiflexion. The tendon can be seen and felt to move under the palpating

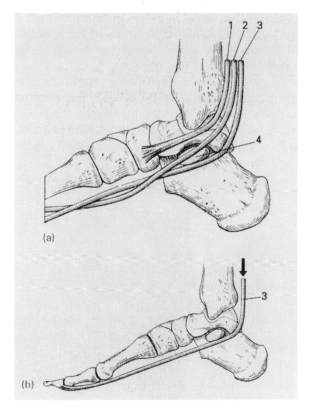

Fig. 6.20 The tendons at the medial malleolus: 1, tibialis posterior; 2, flexor digitorum longus; 3, flexor hallucis longus; 4, sustentaculum tali.

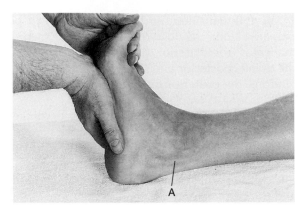

Fig. 6.21 Visualization of the flexor hallucis longus.

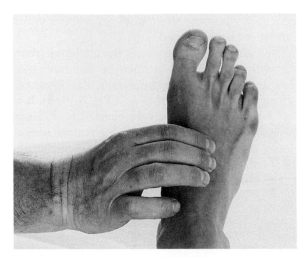

Fig. 6.23 Palpation of the dorsalis pedis artery.

finger when a passive dorsiflexion movement is imposed on the big toe.

DORSAL

The medial and lateral malleoli are easily palpated. A horizontal line drawn 2 cm proximal to the tip of the lateral malleolus and 1 cm proximal to the tip of the medial malleolus closely delineates the inferior tibial border.

During a resisted dorsiflexion, the tendons of the tibialis anterior (Fig. 6.22, A), the extensor hallucis longus (B) and the extensor digitorum longus (C) are visible. The tendon of the peroneus tertius may be visible as the most lateral tendon

running just distally to the sinus tarsi and joining the fifth metatarsal bone.

The pulse of the dorsalis pedis artery can be felt between the tendons of the extensor hallucis longus and the extensor digitorum longus (Fig. 6.23). In about 5% of the population the artery is very thin or even absent.

FUNCTIONAL EXAMINATION OF ANKLE AND FOOT

Introduction/general remarks

The ankle and foot are examined with the subject in the supine lying position.

The ankle and foot are very difficult to examine because a great number of strong and rather stiff structures are condensed into a small volume. To test each structure in turn without the help of a lever is a very difficult task and demands a great technical ability.

The different 'joints' to examine are:

- the ankle joint
- the subtalar joint
- the 'midtarsal joints': the whole middle structure of the foot, though consisting of several bones and joints, functionally acts as one integrated structure and is therefore examined as one 'midtarsal joint'.

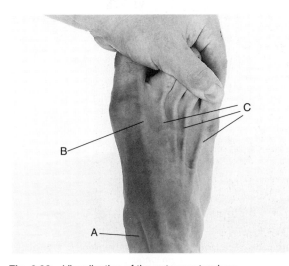

Fig. 6.22 Visualization of the extensor tendons.

The action of the contractile structures of the ankle and foot have an influence on all the different joints.

PASSIVE TESTS OF THE ANKLE JOINT

Passive plantar flexion

Positioning. The subject lies supine with the leg on the couch and the ankle in neutral position. The examiner is distal to the foot. One hand supports the heel, the other is at the dorsum of the foot.

Procedure. A simultaneous movement of both hands pulls and pushes the ankle into plantar flexion (Fig. 6.24).

Common mistakes. None.

Normal functional anatomy:
- *Range*: the dorsal aspect of the foot falls into line with the tibia
- *End-feel*: hard ligamentous

- *Limiting structures*:
  – the engagement of the heel via the Achilles tendon against the back of the tibia
  – anterior tibiotalar ligament.

Common pathological situations:
- Limitation of plantar flexion is usually caused by an articular lesion.
- Anterior pain in combination with a normal end-feel indicates stretching of anterior structures (capsule, tendons of dorsiflexors, anterior tibiotalar and anterior talofibular ligaments).
- Posterior pain is elicited when a pathological structure is painfully squeezed between tibia and calcaneus (bursa, insertion of Achilles tendon, periostitis).

Passive dorsiflexion

Positioning. The ankle is in neutral position with the heel resting on the couch. The knee is slightly flexed. The examiner is distal to the foot. He places one hand at the plantar aspect of the forefoot. The other hand is at the back of the heel.

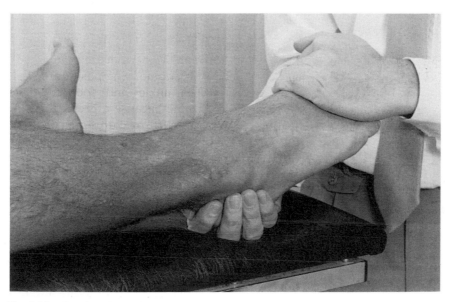

Fig. 6.24 Passive plantar flexion.

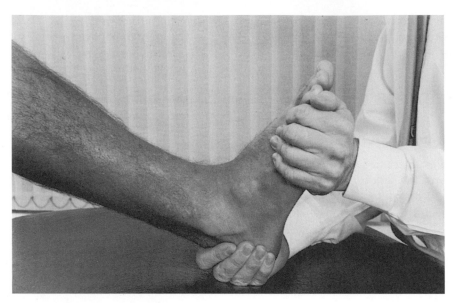

Fig. 6.25 Passive dorsiflexion.

Procedure. Move the foot in the dorsal direction, meanwhile keeping the knee in a slightly flexed position (Fig. 6.25).

Common mistakes. None.

Normal functional anatomy:
- *Range*: the angle between the dorsum of the foot and the tibia can be reduced to less than 90°
- *End-feel*: hard ligamentous
- *Limiting structures*:
  - the posterior capsule
  - posterior talofibular ligament
  - posterior fibres of the deltoid ligament
  - anterior engagement of talar neck and anterior margin of tibial surface.

Common pathological situations:
- Limitation of dorsiflexion is caused by articular lesions or by short calf muscles.
- Posterior pain indicates stretching of posterior structures (capsule or tendons of plantiflexors).
- Anterior pain is elicited when a pathological structure is painfully squeezed between tibia

and talus (anterior periostitis or nipping of post-traumatic fibrosis).

PASSIVE TESTS OF THE SUBTALAR JOINT
Varus movement

Positioning. The heel rests on the couch with the knee slightly flexed and the ankle in neutral position. The examiner is distal to the foot and grasps the heel between the clasped hands. In order to avoid movements in the ankle joint the talus is stabilized between tibial and fibular malleoli. This is achieved by traction on the heel and through a slight pressure with the trunk against the patient's forefoot.

Procedure. Swing the upper half of the body inwards (Fig. 6.26).

Common mistakes:
- Full dorsiflexion is lost.
- Uncomfortable pressure is exerted on the calcaneus.

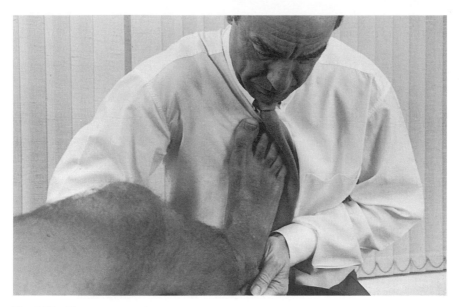

Fig. 6.26   Varus movement.

Normal functional anatomy:
- *Range*: 15–30°
- *End-feel*: ligamentous
- *Limiting structures*:
  - calcaneofibular ligament
  - talocalcanean interosseus ligament
  - joint capsule
  - posterior fibres of the deltoid ligament.

Common pathological situations:
- A progressive limitation of varus indicates a capsular lesion of the subtalar joint. In significant arthritis varus is completely lost by a spasm of the peronei.
- Lateral pain at full range may be indicative of a sprain of the calcaneofibular ligament.

Valgus movement

Positioning. The heel rests on the couch, the knee is slightly flexed and the ankle in neutral position. The examiner is distal to the foot and grasps the heel between the clasped hands. In order to avoid movements in the ankle joint the talus is stabilized between tibial and fibular malleoli. This is achieved by traction on the heel and through a slight pressure with the trunk against the patient's forefoot.

Procedure. Swing the upper half of the body outwards (Fig. 6.27).

Common mistakes:
- Full dorsiflexion is lost.
- Uncomfortable pressure is exerted on the calcaneus.

Normal functional anatomy:
- *Range*: 10–15°
- *End-feel*: ligamentous
- *Limiting structures*:
  - posterior fibres of the deltoid ligament
  - talocalcanean interosseus ligament
  - joint capsule.

Common pathological situations. Medial pain may indicate a lesion of the deltoid ligament.

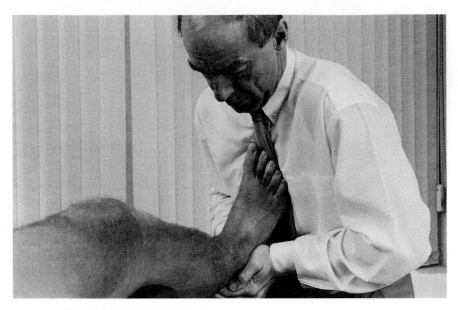

Fig. 6.27 Valgus movement.

PASSIVE TESTS OF THE MIDTARSAL JOINTS

Remarks
- Because the middle segment of the foot consists of several bones and joints it is very difficult to assess isolated movements. Therefore the whole middle segment is considered as one integrated structure.
- Movements are possible in three directions but owing to anatomical characteristics plantar flexion is always accompanied by some adduction, and dorsiflexion by some abduction.
- The positioning for all the midtarsal movements is the same.

Positioning for testing the midtarsal mobility. The subject lies supine with an extended knee and the foot in neutral position. The examiner is distal to the foot. His contralateral hand encircles the heel and carries it. The hand also pulls on the heel and forces it into full valgus. The ipsilateral hand encircles the forefoot, thumb under the metatarsal heads and fingers at the dorsum of the metatarsal shafts.

In this position both ankle and subtalar joints are fully stabilized:
- The traction forces the talus into a dorsiflexed position between the two malleoli.
- The valgus position fixes the subtalar joint.

Common pathological situations for the midtarsal tests:
- Limitation may indicate arthritis or arthrosis.
- Painful movement with an excessive range is typical for the beginning of a midtarsal strain.
- Localized pain indicates a local ligamentous lesion or local periostitis.

Passive dorsiflexion (Fig. 6.28)

Procedure. Press the thumb upwards by a supination of the wrist.

Common mistakes. The ankle and subtalar joints are not stabilized.

Normal functional anatomy:
- *Range*: 10–15°
- *End-feel*: hard ligamentous

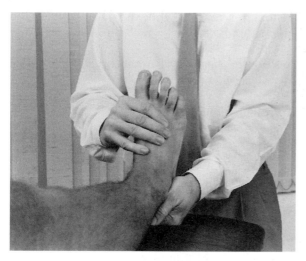

Fig. 6.28   Passive dorsiflexion.

- *Limiting structures*:
  - plantar midtarsal ligaments
  - plantar fascia.

Passive plantar flexion (Fig. 6.29)

Procedure: Press the fingers downwards by a pronation of the wrist.

Common mistakes. The ankle and subtalar joints are not stabilized.

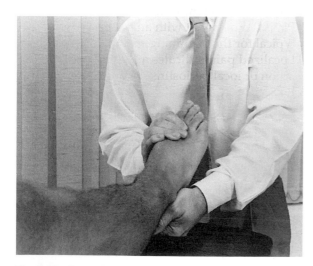

Fig. 6.29   Passive plantar flexion.

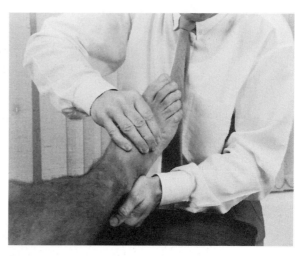

Fig. 6.30   Passive abduction.

Normal functional anatomy:
- *Range*: 10–15°
- *End-feel*: hard ligamentous
- *Limiting structures*: dorsal midtarsal ligaments.

Passive abduction (Fig. 6.30)

Procedure. Perform the abduction movement in the wrist: the web of the thumb presses the medial aspect of the first metatarsal bone in a lateral direction; meanwhile the fingertips provide counter-pressure at the outer side of the forefoot.

Common mistakes. The ankle and subtalar joints are not stabilized.

Normal functional anatomy:
- *Range*: 10–15°
- *End-feel*: hard ligamentous
- *Limiting structures*: medial and inferior midtarsal ligaments.

Passive adduction (Fig. 6.31)

Procedure. Perform the adduction movement in the wrist: the fingertips pull the outer side of the forefoot in a medial direction; meanwhile the fifth metacarpal bone provides counter-pressure.

Common mistakes. The ankle and subtalar joints are not stabilized.

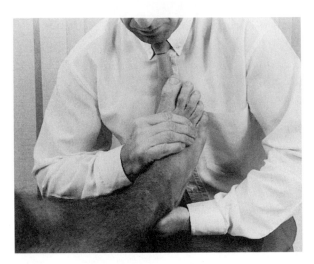

Fig. 6.31 Passive adduction.

Normal functional anatomy:
- *Range*: 10–15°
- *End-feel*: hard ligamentous
- *Limiting structures*: lateral midtarsal ligaments.

Passive pronation (Fig. 6.32)

Procedure. Perform an adduction movement in the shoulder: the hand pulls the inner side of the foot downwards while the thumb pushes the outer side upwards.

Common mistakes. The ankle and subtalar joints are not stabilized.

Normal functional anatomy:
- *Range*: 30–60°
- *End-feel*: soft ligamentous
- *Limiting structures*: medial and dorsal midtarsal ligaments.

Passive supination (Fig. 6.33)

Procedure. Perform an abduction movement in the shoulder: the thumb pulls the inner side of the foot upwards while the fingers push the outer side downwards.

Common mistakes. The ankle and subtalar joints are not stabilized.

Normal functional anatomy:
- *Range*: 45–90°
- *End-feel*: soft ligamentous
- *Limiting structures*: medial and lateral midtarsal ligaments.

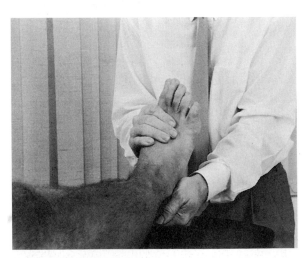

Fig. 6.32 Passive pronation.

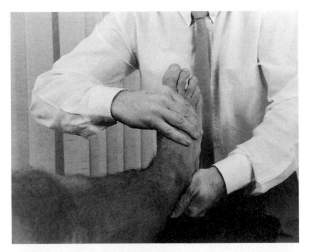

Fig. 6.33 Passive supination.

MAXIMAL ISOMETRIC CONTRACTIONS OF THE FOOT

Resisted dorsiflexion of the foot

Positioning. The subject lies supine with the knee extended and the foot in neutral position. The examiner is distal to the foot. Both hands are placed at the dorsum of the forefoot.

Procedure. Ask the patient to extend the foot (Fig. 6.34).

Common mistakes. None.

Anatomical structures tested:

Muscle function:
• Tibialis anterior
• Extensor hallucis longus
• Extensor digitorum longus
• Peroneus tertius.

Neural function:

Muscle	Innervation	
	Peripheral	Spinal
Tibialis anterior	Deep peroneal	L4, (L5)
Extensor hallucis longus	Deep peroneal	L4, L5
Extensor digitorum longus	Deep peroneal	L4, L5
Peroneus tertius	Deep peroneal	L4, L5

Resisted plantar flexion of the foot

Positioning. The patient lies supine with the knee extended and the foot in neutral position. The examiner is distal to the foot. One fist is placed under the metatarsal heads while the other hand stabilizes the distal end of the leg just proximal to the malleoli.

Procedure. Ask the subject to plantar flex the foot (Fig. 6.35).

Common mistakes. None.

Anatomical structures tested:

Muscle function:
• Triceps surae
• Tibialis posterior
• Flexor hallucis longus
• Flexor digitorum longus
• Peronei longus et brevis.

Neural function:

Muscle	Innervation	
	Peripheral	Spinal
Triceps surae	Tibial	S1–S2
Tibialis posterior	Tibial	L4/L5, S1
Flexor hallucis longus	Tibial	L5, S1
Flexor digitorum longus	Tibial	L5, S1
Peronei longus et brevis	Superficial peroneal	L5, S1

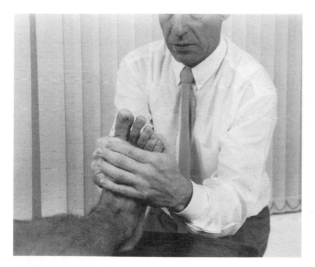

Fig. 6.34   Resisted dorsiflexion.

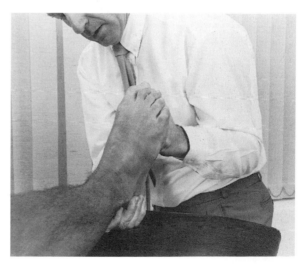

Fig. 6.35   Resisted plantar flexion.

Resisted eversion of the foot

Positioning. The patient lies supine with the knee extended and the foot in neutral position. The examiner is distal to the foot. His ipsilateral hand is placed at the medial and distal end of the leg just above the medial malleolus. The contra-lateral hand is pronated and placed against the lateral border of the foot.

Procedure. Ask the subject to push with the outer side of the foot against the resisting hand (Fig. 6.36).

Common mistakes. The leg is not enough stabilized and an external rotation in the hip rather than an eversion movement in the foot is performed.

Anatomical structures tested:

Muscle function:
- Peroneus longus
- Peroneus brevis
- Peroneus tertius
- Extensor digitorum longus.

Neural function:

Muscle	Innervation	
	Peripheral	Spinal
Peronei longus et brevis	Superficial peroneal	L5, S1
Extensor digitorum longus	Deep peroneal	L4, L5
Peroneus tertius	Deep peroneal	L4, L5

Resisted inversion of the foot

Positioning. The patient lies supine with the knee extended and the foot in neutral position. The examiner is distal to the foot. The contra-lateral hand is placed at the lateral and distal end of the leg just above the lateral malleolus. The ipsilateral hand is placed against the medial border of the foot.

Procedure. Ask the subject to press the inner side of the foot against the resisting hand (Fig. 6.37).

Common mistakes. The leg is not properly stabilized and an internal rotation in the hip rather than an inversion movement at the foot is performed.

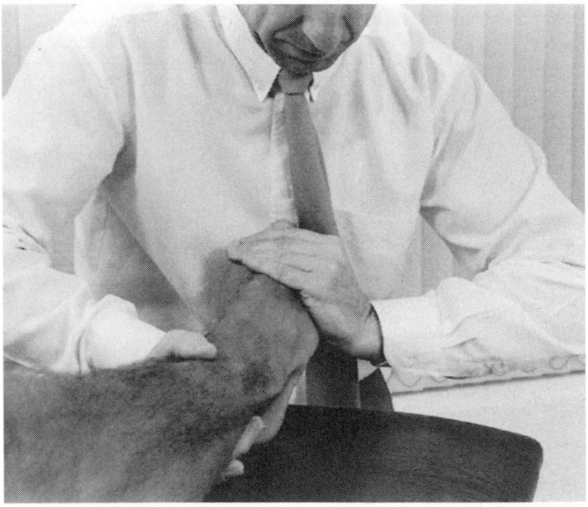

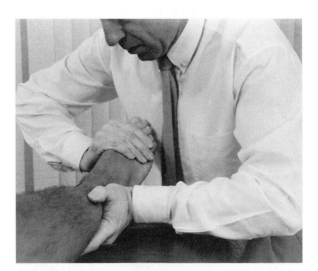

Fig. 6.36 Resisted eversion.

Fig. 6.37 Resisted inversion.

Anatomical structures tested:

Muscle function:
- Tibialis posterior
- Tibialis anterior
- Flexor hallucis longus
- Extensor hallucis longus
- Triceps surae.

Neural function:

Muscle	Innervation	
	Peripheral	Spinal
Tibialis posterior	Tibial	L4/L5, S1
Tibialis anterior	Deep peroneal	L4, (L5)
Flexor hallucis longus	Tibial	L5, S1
Extensor hallucis longus	Deep peroneal	L4, L5
Triceps surae	Tibial	S1–S2

SPECIFIC TESTS

Combined plantar flexion–inversion

Significance. This movement brings all the lateral structures of ankle and foot under stretch and is therefore an extremely important test in sprained ankles.

Positioning. The heel rests on the couch, the knee is slightly flexed and the ankle is in neutral position. The examiner is distal to the foot. His ipsilateral hand fixes the leg at the distal and medial side. The contralateral hand is placed on the midfoot, so that the heel of the hand rests at the fifth metacarpal bone and the fingers encircle the medial border.

Procedure. Stabilize the leg with the ipsilateral hand. Press the foot downwards and inwards with the heel of the contralateral hand. Meanwhile perform a supination movement by an upwards pulling of the fingers (Fig. 6.38).

Common mistakes:
- The lower leg is not sufficiently stabilized.
- Plantar flexion is lost.
- Supination is not conducted to the end.
- Painful pinching of the forefoot occurs.

Normal functional anatomy:
- *Range*: 60–120° angle between forefoot and lower leg
- *End feel*: soft ligamentous
- *Limiting structures*:
  - anterior talofibular ligament
  - lateral and dorsal calcaneocuboid ligaments
  - capsule of the cuboid–fifth metatarsal joint
  - peronei longus and brevis tendons
  - extensor digitorum longus tendons.

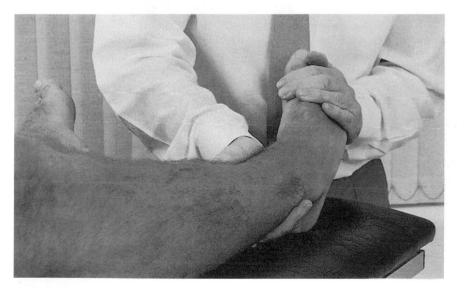

Fig. 6.38 Combined plantar flexion–inversion.

Common pathological situations:
- This movement is extremely painful in ankle sprains.
- Excessive range is noted in total rupture of the anterior talofibular ligament.
- In chronic ankle sprains with ligamentous adhesions there is slight limitation with a tougher end-feel.
- Marked limitation with a spastic end-feel is typical for a subtalar arthritis.

Combined plantar flexion–eversion

Significance. This movement stretches all the medial ligaments of the ankle.

Positioning. The heel rests on the couch, the knee is slightly flexed and the ankle is in neutral position. The examiner is distal to the foot. His contralateral hand fixes the leg at the distal and lateral side. The ipsilateral hand encircles the midfoot with the heel lying on the first metatarsal bone and the fingers encircling the lateral border.

Procedure. Stabilize the leg with the contralateral hand. Press the foot downwards and outwards with the heel of the ipsilateral hand. Meanwhile perform a pronation by an upwards pulling of the fingers (Fig. 6.39).

Common mistakes.
- The lower leg is not stabilized.
- Plantar flexion is lost.
- Pronation is not performed.
- Painful pinching of the forefoot occurs.

Normal functional anatomy:
- *Range*: 15–45°
- *End-feel*: ligamentous
- *Limiting structures*:
  - anterior part of the deltoid ligament
  - calcaneonavicular ligament
  - capsules of the medial midtarsal joints
  - tendon of the tibialis anterior.

Common pathological situations:
- Medial pain may be caused by a lesion of the anterior portion of the deltoid ligament or by a tendinitis of the tibialis posterior.
- Lateral pain may indicate a painful squeezing of the posterior talofibular ligament.

Anterior drawer test

Significance. This is a specific test for the integrity of the anterior talofibular ligament.

Positioning. The subject lies supine and relaxed with the knee flexed to 90°. The heel rests on

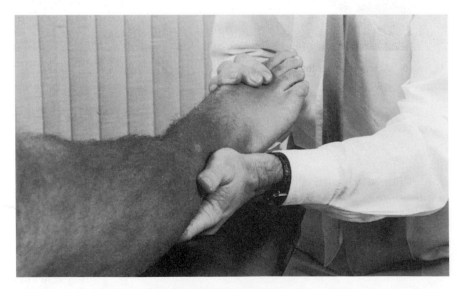

Fig. 6.39 Combined plantar flexion–eversion.

the couch and the foot is in slight plantar flexion. The examiner stands at the opposite side of the foot, level with it. One hand stabilizes the lower leg while the other is placed at the lateral border of the foot.

Procedure. Stabilize the lower leg. Try to move the foot forwards in a medial direction (Fig. 6.40).

Common mistakes:
- The lower leg is not stabilized.
- There is too much plantar flexion at the ankle joint.

Normal functional anatomy:
- *Range*: none
- *End-feel*: ligamentous
- *Limiting structure*: anterior talofibular ligament.

Common pathological situations. The movement is only possible if the anterior talofibular ligament is ruptured or elongated. Movement is indicated by a forwards shift of the lateral margin of the trochlea tali in relation to the lateral malleolus (Fig. 6.41).

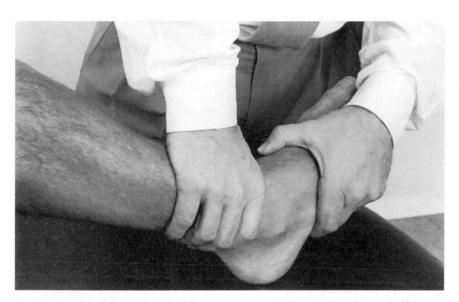

Fig. 6.40 Anterior drawer test.

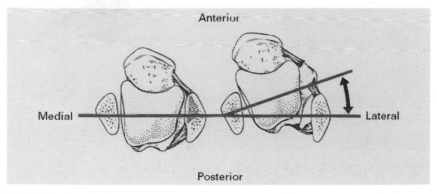

Fig. 6.41 Anterior drawer test.

Combined dorsiflexion–eversion

Significance. This is a specific test to demonstrate anterior periostitis of the fibula.

Positioning. The knee is slightly flexed and the ankle in neutral position. The examiner is distal to the foot. His ipsilateral hand supports the heel and the contralateral hand is placed against the plantar and lateral side of the foot.

Procedure. Press the foot upwards and outwards with the heel of the contralateral hand until the end-feel is ascertained (Fig. 6.42).

Common mistakes. The movement is not executed firmly enough.

Common pathological situations. Lateral pain indicates the existence of periostitis of the inferior border of the fibula. Alternatively the pain is caused by impingement of a thickened, hypertrophied talofibular ligament.

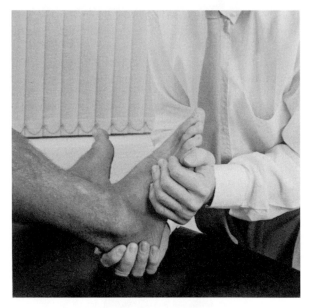

Fig. 6.42   Combined dorsiflexion–eversion.

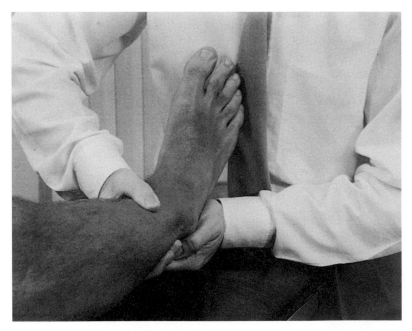

Fig. 6.43   Strong varus movement at the ankle.

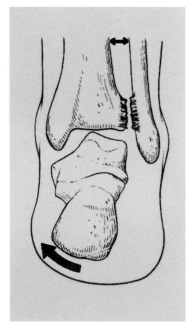

Strong varus movement at the ankle

Significance. This movement tests the integrity of the strong distal tibiofibular ligaments.

Positioning. The ankle is in neutral position and the knee extended. The examiner is distal to the foot. The ipsilateral hand fixes the leg at the inner side, just above the ankle. The contralateral hand grasps the foot at the heel.

Procedure. Force the heel with a strong and quick thrust into varus (Fig. 6.43).

Common mistakes. The movement is not executed firmly enough.

Common pathological situations:
- When there is ligamentous rupture or laxity of the distal tibiofibular ligaments, the fibula can be pressed outwards, a circumstance that is detected by a palpable click when the tibia and the fibula engage after their momentary separation.
- In a total rupture of the anterior talofibular or the calcaneofibular ligaments, this test will also show laxity.

Index

Also by the same authors and published by Harcourt Brace:

L. Ombregt, P. Bisschop, H. J. ter Veer, T. Van de Velde:
A System of Orthopaedic Medicine

A series of CD-roms in orthopedic medicine is being produced by Dr L. Ombregt, Kanegemstraat 170, 8700 Kanegem-Tielt, Belgium.

To order copies and for further details see:

http://ourworld.compuserve.com/homepages/lombregt/index.htm

Please note that this is the author's private production and copies cannot be ordered from Harcourt Brace.